Repurposed Drugs - Current State and Future Perspectives

Edited by Seçkin Engin

Published in London, United Kingdom

Repurposed Drugs - Current State and Future Perspectives
http://dx.doi.org/10.5772/intechopen.1003317
Edited by Seçkin Engin

Contributors
Aaiza Munir, Adam Frymoyer, Annette Bakker, Ashok Kumar Tiwari, Bharti Sapra, D. Wade Clapp, Durga Prasad Beda, Gatadi Srikanth, Hui Bai, Iqra Safdar, Jaishri Blakeley, James Gusella, Jing Wang, Kailen Mark, Kareti Srinivasa Rao, Kathleen M. Sakamoto, Maah Rukh Zahid, Marc Ferrer, Namrata Patel, Niggula Praveen Kumar, Norman Lacayo, Om Silakari, Paranthaman Subash, Rabia Zafar, Saad Serfraz, Scott Plotkin, Seçkin Engin, Shama Parveen, Siming Kong, Song He, Sulekha Khute, Xiaochen Bo, Yunfang Wang

First published in London, United Kingdom, 2025 by IntechOpen
IntechOpen is the global imprint of INTECHOPEN LIMITED, registered in England and Wales, registration number: 11086078, 167-169 Great Portland Street, London, W1W 5PF, United Kingdom

For EU product safety concerns: IN TECH d.o.o., Prolaz Marije Krucifikse Kozulić 3, 51000 Rijeka, Croatia, info@intechopen.com or visit our website at intechopen.com.

British Library Cataloguing-in-Publication Data
A catalogue record for this book is available from the British Library

Repurposed Drugs - Current State and Future Perspectives
Edited by Seçkin Engin
p. cm.

This title is part of the Pharmaceutical Science Book Series, Volume 9
Topic: Drug Discovery and Delivery
Series Editor: Rosario Pignatello
Topic Editor: Marilena Vlachou

Print ISBN 978-0-85014-775-9
Online ISBN 978-0-85014-774-2
eBook (PDF) ISBN 978-0-85014-776-6
ISSN 3033-3318

If disposing of this product, please recycle the paper responsibly.

IntechOpen Book Series

Pharmaceutical Science

Volume 9

Aims and Scope of the Series

Pharmaceutical science focuses on the design, synthesis, formulation, targeting, distribution, safety, and efficacy of active compounds as potential therapeutics. It is a large interdisciplinary discipline that aims to integrate the basic principles of physical and organic chemistry, biochemistry, biology, and engineering to discover, develop, and characterize active compounds and to optimize the formulation and delivery of drugs in the body for offering new and improved safe and efficacious therapies against human diseases. The research areas covered by the pharmaceutical sciences range from medicinal chemistry and pharmaceutical technology to pharmacology and toxicology, which represent the preliminary phases of drug development. Medicinal chemistry involves the design and synthesis of pharmaceuticals as well as the isolation of active agents from natural sources. Computer-aided strategies are increasingly involved in this drug discovery process. Pharmaceutics is a multidisciplinary science that examines the relationships between drug formulation, delivery, distribution, and clinical outcomes. Modern clinical approaches are increasingly relying on controlled release strategies and drug delivery and targeting systems, including nanotechnological platforms (nanomedicine). Pharmacology is the science of drug action in biological systems. Pharmacologists also make drugs as tools to explore aspects of cell and tissue functions. Toxicology is the study of the adverse effects of active agents on living organisms and the ecosystem, including the prevention and amelioration of such adverse effects. This book series includes volumes on Drug Discovery, Delivery, and Pharmacology. Their overall aim is to present the latest research in the whole path of drug discovery and development from different points of view of this multidisciplinary and dynamic field.

Meet the Series Editor

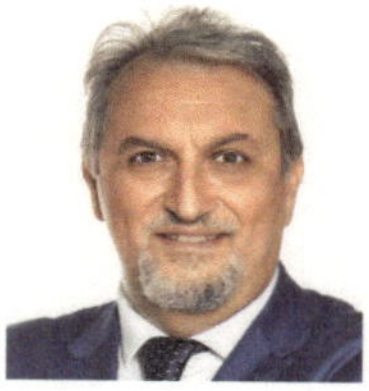

Prof. Rosario Pignatello is a Full Professor of Pharmaceutical Technology and Legislation at the University of Catania, Italy. He is the Director of the Department of Drug and Health Sciences. He has nearly 30 years of experience in the research and development of innovative formulations for the controlled release and targeting of bioactive molecules, through chemical approaches as well as nanotechnological carriers, aimed at treating different disorders. Prof. Pignatello has coauthored about 180 papers and edited a series of textbooks on biomaterials and their application in medicine. The main areas of his research are polymeric and lipid-based micro- and nanoparticles as modified drug delivery systems; vesicular nanocarriers (liposomes, micelles); lipophilic prodrugs and conjugates; synthesis and evaluation of new polymeric biomaterials for drug delivery and tissue regeneration. In particular, Prof. Pignatello works actively in the field of ocular drug delivery, leading the Research Centre for Ocular Nanotechnology, within the NANOMED Centre (Centre for Nanomedicine and Pharmaceutical Nanotechnology) at the University of Catania.

Meet the Volume Editor

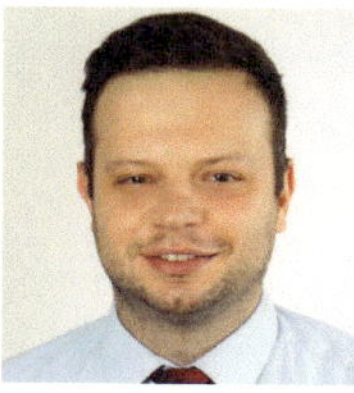

Seçkin Engin received his BS in Pharmacy (2013) from Gazi University in Türkiye and a Ph.D. in Pharmacology (2020) from the Health Sciences Institute of Karadeniz Technical University in Türkiye. He currently works as a full-time researcher and lecturer in the Department of Pharmacology at the Faculty of Pharmacy at the Karadeniz Technical University. He has published multiple scientific papers and book chapters as the lead author in peer-reviewed international journals. He is also a journal peer reviewer and a member of the editorial boards of journals. His research interests include smooth muscle pharmacology and urogenital system pharmacology, which are focused on identifying novel drugs or drugs repurposing for cystitis and diabetic urological complications such as erectile dysfunction and diabetic cystopathy.

Contents

Preface

Drug repurposing or repositioning is defined as the strategy of drug development that identifies novel therapeutic uses that are outside the scope of the original medical indication for already available drugs. In recent years, drug repurposing has received remarkable global interest, accelerating the preclinical process and reducing time and cost, thus providing the high potential to overcome the challenges of traditional drug discovery. Owing to its superior advantages, drug repurposing is currently considered the lead strategy for drug development in rare diseases and cancers, offering opportunities to meet the urgent need for therapeutic options. Moreover, artificial intelligence and machine learning techniques in drug repurposing have particularly gained attention, making it one of the most popular topics in drug development. Due to its continuously growing and dynamic nature, it is an increasing concern to closely track recent developments in drug repurposing. Thus, this book offers a comprehensive update on the current state and future perspectives of repurposed drugs. After an introductory chapter that presents the background and context of the subject, this book includes chapters that summarise hot topics surrounding the subject as follows:

Chapter 1: "Introductory Chapter: Repurposed Drugs - Current State and Future Perspectives"

Chapter 2: "Repurposed Drugs: Current Trends in Drug Discovery"

Chapter 3: "Drug Repositioning in the AI-Driven Era: Data, Approaches, and Challenges"

Chapter 4: "Advantages, Challenges, and Impact of Drug Repurposing for Cancer Treatment"

Chapter 5: "Computational Drug Repositioning Method Applied to Lung Cancer"

Chapter 6: "Repurposing Niclosamide for Treatment of Acute Myeloid Leukemia and Other Diseases"

Chapter 7: "Unlocking Brigatinib's Potential: A Remarkable Case of Drug Repurposing in NF2-SWN"

Chapter 8: "Design Strategies for Smart Hydrogels: From Concept to Application"

Written by experts in the field, this book is essential reading to all scientists involved in drug discovery and development, clinicians, healthcare professionals, and students.

I want to thank all the authors for their valuable contributions and great efforts in providing this important scientific book.

Seçkin Engin, Ph.D.
Faculty of Pharmacy,
Department of Pharmacology,
Karadeniz Technical University,
Trabzon, Türkiye

Section 1

General Concepts

Chapter 1

Introductory Chapter: Repurposed Drugs – Current State and Future Perspectives

Seçkin Engin

1. Introduction

Traditional de novo drug discovery is known to be a long, expensive, and costly process, from discovering compounds to its approval, taking approximately 12–17 years and requiring large investments of more than $2 billion per new drug, and unfortunately, most of the new drug candidates fail during this process making it a risky business [1, 2]. The high cost of traditional drug discovery currently represents a major concern for the global pharmaceutical industry to address unmet medical needs for various diseases. To overcome these challenges, tremendous effort has still been devoted to developing alternative approaches for drug discovery by academia, pharmaceutical companies, and regulators [3, 4].

Drug repurposing or repositioning (also called reprofiling, redirecting, switching, etc.) is a recent concept of drug discovery and development to identify novel therapeutic uses for approved drugs different from the original indication, which is a growing trend in the pharmaceutical industry [5]. Drug repurposing offers opportunities for the drug discovery process to lower the risk of failure and reduce cost and time frame. Because the repurposed drugs have completed preclinical testing and safety assessment, the relevant drug information already exists, promoting accelerated drug development. Owing to drug repurposing, many therapeutics have been introduced in the market for several diseases [5, 6]. Besides its many advantages, drug repurposing also faces some limitations. In most cases, repurposed drugs are currently off-patent, so they do not receive appreciated commercial interest from pharmaceutical companies. In addition, repurposed drugs could not be effective in monotherapy, and thus higher doses, prolonged treatment periods, and/or different formulations may be necessary to obtain sufficient efficacy for the novel use compared with the original indication, which requires further investigation [7, 8]. Remarkable advances in technology and science have recently made various computational methods available with the help of artificial intelligence for the identification of repurposable drug candidates [9].

2. Trends in drug repurposing

Cancer now stands out as the leading cause of death worldwide. Although various anticancer drugs currently exist, they are commonly associated with insufficient efficacy and/or tolerability, pointing out a major challenge in oncology. Thus, drug repurposing has gained considerable interest in seeking a novel anticancer drug in the past decade, making it a hot topic in oncology drug development [10]. Until now, several lines of evidence demonstrate the potential anticancer effects of approved noncancer drugs. Aspirin can be considered one of the oldest repurposed drugs. Although initially developed as an analgesic, aspirin at low doses was repurposed as an antiplatelet drug in the 1980s. Recently, aspirin has also been recommended to prevent the development of many cancers, particularly colorectal cancer. As another example of a repurposed drug in cancer, thalidomide, an antiemetic drug, was withdrawn in 1962 because of its teratogenicity. Then, thalidomide was repurposed for multiple myeloma in 2006 due to its antiangiogenic activity, providing the new life for thalidomide in clinical use [11]. In recent years, drug repurposing in cancer has prominently accelerated owing to great advances in disease biology and omics coupled with artificial intelligence methods [12].

Rare diseases represent a unique group of disorders seen in a small percentage of the population, affecting more than 350 million patients globally. Nearly 7000 rare diseases are currently identified, and a majority of them still lack specific treatment to cure [13]. Only fewer than 6% of all rare diseases have licensed drugs, emphasizing the high demand for drug development. Now, most patients with rare diseases can only be symptomatically treated with drugs to improve their quality of life. Hence, drug repurposing is an attractive strategy to develop efficient treatment options for rare diseases [13, 14]. Tretinoin, a derivative of vitamin A, was first used topically in the treatment of acne vulgaris. In 1995, an oral capsule of tretinoin was approved by the FDA for induction of remission in acute promyelocytic leukemia, a rare disease. Sildenafil and tadalafil are phosphodiesterase PDE5 inhibitors widely used for erectile dysfunction, and both were then approved for pulmonary arterial hypertension, which is a rare and progressive lung disease [14]. NF2-related schwannomatosis (NF2-SWN) is a rare genetic disorder with no FDA-approved treatments, characterized by the growth of benign tumors in the nervous system leading to tinnitus, hearing loss, and balance dysfunction [15]. Briganitib is a small molecule inhibitor of anaplastic lymphoma kinase (ALK) approved by the FDA for adult patients with ALK-positive metastatic non-small cell lung cancer. In recent studies, brigatinib has been reported to show promising outcomes, which could be repurposed for NF2-SWN [16].

Niclosamide is a widely used FDA-approved oral antihelminthic drug to treat parasitic infections. However, recent studies have reported that niclosamide may have a broad spectrum of therapeutic effects against various clinical conditions, including cancer, bacterial and viral infection, metabolic diseases, endometriosis, neuropathic pain, rheumatoid arthritis, sclerodermatous graft-versus-host disease, and systemic sclerosis [17]. Due to its complex mechanisms of actions interfering with multiple signaling pathways such as Wnt/β-catenin, mTORC1, STAT3, NF-κB, and Notch signaling, niclosamide is one of the most attractive repurposed drugs that are still under intensive investigation [17, 18].

Pharmaceutical formulation of the approved drugs is an important process while repurposing drugs for novel indications. As mentioned, the new use of the drug can require different dosage forms of formulation. Therefore, recent advances in drug delivery systems should also be taken into consideration to prepare more appropriate dosage forms for new uses.

In summary, drug repurposing has led to remarkable progress in drug development to meet medication needs, and it is a highly preferred strategy of drug development, especially for cancer and rare diseases, by providing reduced cost and a shortened time frame. Hence, repurposed drugs are considered to become more widespread as potential therapeutics owing to artificial intelligence-driven computational methods in the near future.

Author details

Seçkin Engin
Department of Pharmacology, Faculty of Pharmacy, Karadeniz Technical University, Trabzon, Turkey

*Address all correspondence to: seckinengin@ktu.edu.tr

References

[1] Tobinick EL. The value of drug repositioning in the current pharmaceutical market. Drug News & Perspectives. 2009;**22**(2):119-125. DOI: 10.1358/dnp.2009.22.2.1303818

[2] Hua Y, Dai X, Xu Y, Xing G, Liu H, Lu T, et al. Drug repositioning: Progress and challenges in drug discovery for various diseases. European Journal of Medicinal Chemistry. 2022;**234**:114239. DOI: 10.1016/j.ejmech.2022.114239

[3] Pushpakom S, Iorio F, Eyers PA, Escott KJ, Hopper S, Wells A, et al. Drug repurposing: Progress, challenges and recommendations. Nature Reviews Drug Discovery. 2019;**18**(1):41-58. DOI: 10.1038/nrd.2018.168

[4] Oprea T, Mestres J. Drug repurposing: Far beyond new targets for old drugs. The AAPS Journal. 2012;**14**:759-763. DOI: 10.1208/s12248-012-9390-1

[5] Olgen S. A prospective overview of drug repurposing in drug discovery and development. Current Medicinal Chemistry. 2019;**26**(28):5338-5339. DOI: 10.2174/092986732628191025094454

[6] Parvathaneni V, Kulkarni NS, Muth A, Gupta V. Drug repurposing: A promising tool to accelerate the drug discovery process. Drug Discovery Today. 2019;**24**(10):2076-2085. DOI: 10.1016/j.drudis.2019.06.014

[7] Boyer A, Pasquier E, Tomasini P, et al. Drug repurposing in malignant pleural mesothelioma: A breath of fresh air? European Respiratory Review: An Official Journal of the European Respiratory Society. 2018;**27**(147):170098. DOI: 10.1183/16000617.0098-2017

[8] Ahmed K, Shaw HV, Koval A, Katanaev VL. A second WNT for old drugs: Drug repositioning against WNT-dependent cancers. Cancers (Basel). 2016;**8**(7):66. DOI: 10.3390/cancers8070066

[9] Aljofan M, Gaipov A. Drug discovery and development: The role of artificial intelligence in drug repurposing. Future Medicinal Chemistry. 2024;**16**(7):583-585. DOI: 10.4155/fmc-2024-0048

[10] Xia Y, Sun M, Huang H, Jin WL. Drug repurposing for cancer therapy. Signal Transduction and Targeted Therapy. 2024;**9**(1):92. DOI: 10.1038/s41392-024-01808-1

[11] Jourdan JP, Bureau R, Rochais C, Dallemagne P. Drug repositioning: A brief overview. Journal of Pharmacy and Pharmacology. 2020;**72**(9):1145-1151. DOI: 10.1111/jphp.13273

[12] Wieder R, Adam N. Drug repositioning for cancer in the era of AI, big omics, and real-world data. Critical Reviews in Oncology/Hematology. 2022;**175**:103730. DOI: 10.1016/j.critrevonc.2022.103730

[13] Roessler HI, Knoers NVAM, van Haelst MM, van Haaften G. Drug repurposing for rare diseases. Trends in Pharmacological Sciences. 2021;**42**(4):255-267. DOI: 10.1016/j.tips.2021.01.003

[14] Sardana D, Zhu C, Zhang M, Gudivada RC, Yang L, Jegga AG. Drug repositioning for orphan diseases. Briefings in Bioinformatics. 2011;**12**(4):346-356. DOI: 10.1093/bib/bbr021

[15] Kim BH, Chung YH, Woo TG, et al. NF2-related Schwannomatosis (NF2): Molecular insights and therapeutic avenues. International Journal of Molecular Sciences. 2024;**25**(12):6558. DOI: 10.3390/ijms25126558

[16] Plotkin SR, Yohay KH, Nghiemphu PL, et al. Brigatinib in NF2-related schwannomatosis with progressive tumors. New England Journal of Medicine. 2024;**390**(24):2284-2294. DOI: 10.1056/NEJMoa2400985

[17] Chen W, Mook RA Jr, Premont RT, Wang J. Niclosamide: Beyond an antihelminthic drug. Cellular Signalling. 2018;**41**:89-96. DOI: 10.1016/j.cellsig.2017.04.001

[18] Wang Z, Ren J, Du J, Wang H, Liu J, Wang G. Niclosamide as a promising therapeutic player in human cancer and other diseases. International Journal of Molecular Sciences. 2022;**23**(24):16116. DOI: 10.3390/ijms232416116

Chapter 2

Repurposed Drugs: Current Trends in Drug Discovery

Gatadi Srikanth, Durga Prasad Beda and Niggula Praveen Kumar

Abstract

Drug repurposing is a drug discovery strategy that involves identifying new therapeutic uses for existing drugs. Drug repurposing relies on the idea that a limited number of genes or gene products mediate biological processes and that several biological entities—such as transcripts, proteins, and genes—have pleiotropic effects and mediate similar tasks. Recently, drug repurposing has gained attention as a different approach that looks for novel uses for previously approved or rejected commercial medications to address conditions other than those they were designed for. It offers numerous benefits, such as faster development timelines, reduced costs, established safety profiles, and the potential for novel treatments for unmet medical needs. This chapter explains the current trends in drug discovery and future perspectives on repurposed drugs.

Keywords: drug repurposing, repurposed drugs, diseases, drug discovery, future perspectives

1. Introduction

Drug repurposing (DR) is also termed as drug repositioning, drug re-tasking, drug reprofiling, drug rescuing, drug recycling, drug redirection, and therapeutic switching. This drug discovery strategy aims to find new therapeutic uses for previously investigated, already marketed, FDA-approved, old, existing, failed drugs or pro-drugs. The newly developed drugs are then applied to treat diseases other than the original or intended therapeutic use. It entails finding novel therapeutic applications for previously approved, stopped, abandoned, and experimental medications [1–3]. The process of finding new drugs by traditional means is risky, costly, time-consuming, and labor-intensive. It may be a more effective strategy because medication repositioning reduces the high financial cost, longer development time, and higher failure rate associated with traditional drug discovery programs. It has the added benefit of saving up to 5–7 years in average drug development time. In conventional drug discovery programs, failure rates of approximately 45% are linked to safety or toxicity issues. This reduces the likelihood of failure. Around one-third of newly approved treatments are repurposed medications, accounting for 25% of the pharmaceutical industry's yearly income [4–6]. This indicates that the drug repositioning strategy has acquired significant traction recently. Repositioned pharmaceuticals comprise about 30% of US Food and Drug Administration (FDA) approved medications and biologics (vaccines). The pharmaceutical companies estimated the market for repurposed pharmaceuticals to be worth $24.4 billion in 2015, and it is expected to grow to $31.3 billion by 2020. The earliest known instance of drug repositioning dates back to a coincidental finding or observation in the 1920s. More methods for quickening medication repositioning were created after roughly a century of research and development.

The most well-known and effective medications from the DR method include methotrexate, valproic acid, aspirin, minoxidil, thalidomide, and sildenafil [7].

Drug name	Original indication	New indication	Date of approval	Repurposing approach used
Zidovudine	Cancer	HIV/AIDS	1987	*In vitro* screening of compound libraries
Minoxidil	Hypertension	Hair loss	1988	Retrospective analysis (observed hair growth as adverse effect)
Sildenafil	Angina	Erectile dysfunction	1998	Retrospective clinical analysis
Thalidomide	Morning sickness	Erythema nodosum leprosum and multiple myeloma	1998 and 2006	Off-label usage and pharmacological analysis
Celecoxib	Pain and inflammation	Familial adenomatous polyps	2000	Pharmacological analysis
Atomoxetine	Parkinson's disease	ADHD	2002	Pharmacological analysis
Duloxetine	Depression	SUI	2004	Pharmacological analysis
Rituximab	Various cancers	Rheumatoid arthritis	2006	Retrospective clinical analysis (remission of coexisting rheumatoid arthritis in patients with non-Hodgkin lymphoma treated with rituximab)
Raloxifene	Osteoporosis	Breast cancer	2007	Retrospective clinical analysis
Fingolimod	Transplant rejection	MS	2010	Pharmacological and structural analysis
Dapoxetine	Analgesia and depression	Premature ejaculation	2012	Pharmacological analysis
Topiramate	Epilepsy	Obesity	2012	Pharmacological analysis
Ketoconazole	Fungal infections	Cushing syndrome	2014	Pharmacological analysis
Aspirin	Analgesia	Colorectal cancer	2015	Pharmacological analysis Retrospective clinical and Pharmacological analysis

Table 1.
Some of the repurposed drugs according to their year of approval and the approach used.

For instance, sildenafil was first created as a blood pressure-lowering medication. However, Pfizer repurposed it to treat erectile dysfunction and marketed it under the brand name Viagra. As a result, in 2012, it held a market-leading 47% share of the erectile dysfunction drug market, with sales of $2.05 billion worldwide [8]. Thalidomide, a chiral medication that was first marketed as a sedative in certain countries in 1957, was regrettably taken off the market within 4 years because of its well-known association with birth abnormalities resembling seal limbs in children whose mothers took the medication during the first trimester of their pregnancies [9]. However, it was shockingly shown to be effective in treating ENL1 in 1964 and multiple myeloma decades later in 1999. Since then, it has significantly benefited the market for multiple myeloma patients. It has also aided in developing and approving even more successful medications, like lenalidomide (Revlimid, Celgene), which had $8.2 billion in global sales in 2017 [10]. **Table 1** lists additional drugs that have been successfully repurposed, along with the repurposing strategies used. Most of these repurposing strategies have resulted from knowledge of the drug's clinical effectiveness or from retrospective analyses of the pharmacological effect of a drug when prescribed for its original indication.

2. Accelerated drug development process

The potential benefits of drug repurposing compared to de novo drug discovery are diverse; however, drug repurposing predominantly allows for an quickened drug development technique as compared to the classical way for de novo drug development (**Figure 1a**) [11, 12]. Repurposing efforts circumvent many preclinical stages of drug discovery process, since kinetics. and toxicity profiles of the drugs are already familiar [13].

The only requirement for the preclinical stage is the evidence of efficacy for the additional indication in either a cell or animal model since the lead candidate has probably already undergone safety and toxicity testing for the accurate indication. A successful outcome may result in submitting an Investigational New Drug Application to the FDA in the United States. This application is only eligible for the 505(b)(2) process, which permits using data from earlier studies to assess the drug candidate. As a result, the lead candidate can typically skip the lengthy Phase I safety studies and go straight to Phase IIa clinical trials, when safety is evaluated much less rigorously and expensively [14]. A New Drug Application is the result of successful clinical trial outcomes, and the drug that has been repurposed can reach the market (**Figure 1b**). This can lead to shorter development timelines, lower costs, and a decrease in development risks because safety—the main obstacle to drug discovery—is well established. Economically speaking, skipped developmental stages (like Phase I) provide savings of about 15% of the total cost. This implies that the procedure for repurposing pharmaceuticals should take 3–12 years, while *de novo* drug discovery should take 10–17 years [15]. Because important factors like chemical optimization, manufacturing, and formulation are frequently well established and may be ruled out, a quicker path to the clinic is also feasible.

Moreover, drug repurposing can further reduce the costs of developing new therapies when patent protection expires, allowing generic manufacturing. Thus, savings for consumers are vast. These are all benefits when it comes to repurposed drugs; accordingly, several efforts are becoming progressively attractive.

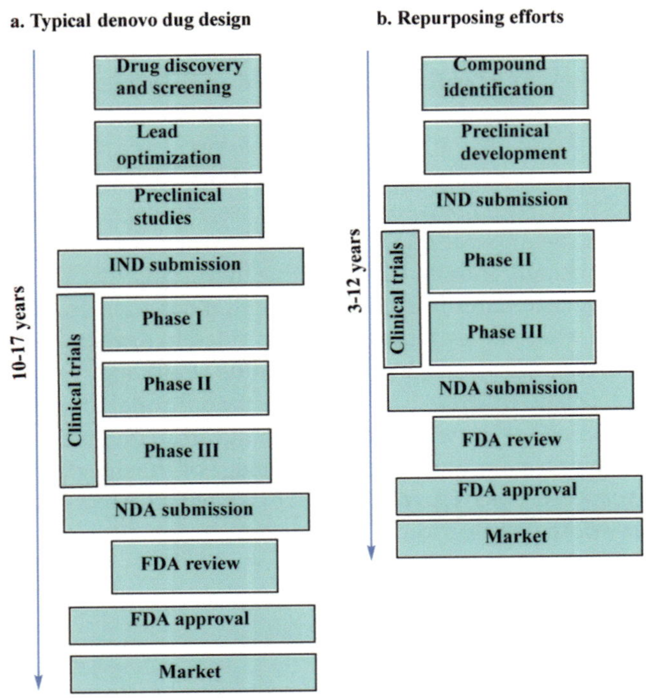

Figure 1.
(a and b) Schematic representation of the regulatory process for licensing conventional versus repurposed compounds.

3. Strategies of drug repurposing

On-target and off-target are the two primary DR techniques (**Figure 2**). On-target DR applies a medication molecule's established pharmacological action to a novel therapeutic application. This approach uses a different disease but the same therapeutic molecule's biological target [16].

For example, an on-target profile is seen in repositioning minoxidil (Rogaine) since the medication operates on the same target while generating two distinct therapeutic effects. From an antihypertensive vasodilator to an anti-hair loss medication, minoxidil transformed. The pharmacological effect of minoxidil, an antihypertensive vasodilator, helps to cure male pattern baldness (androgenic alopecia) by widening blood vessels and activating potassium channels, which increases the amount of blood, oxygen, and nutrients that reach the hair follicles. However, the pharmacological mechanism in the off-target profile needs to be understood. Pharmaceuticals and drug candidates function on novel targets beyond their original intended use for novel therapeutic purposes. As a result, the indicators and the objectives are novel [17]. An excellent illustration of an off-target profile is aspirin (Colsprin). Historically, aspirin has been used as an NSAID to treat a variety of inflammatory and pain conditions. Additionally, it reduces blood coagulation (clot formation) by impeding platelets' ability to function normally (antiplatelet medication). Consequently, it is applied in the management of strokes and heart attacks. There have also been reports of aspirin being used in a novel way to treat prostate cancer.

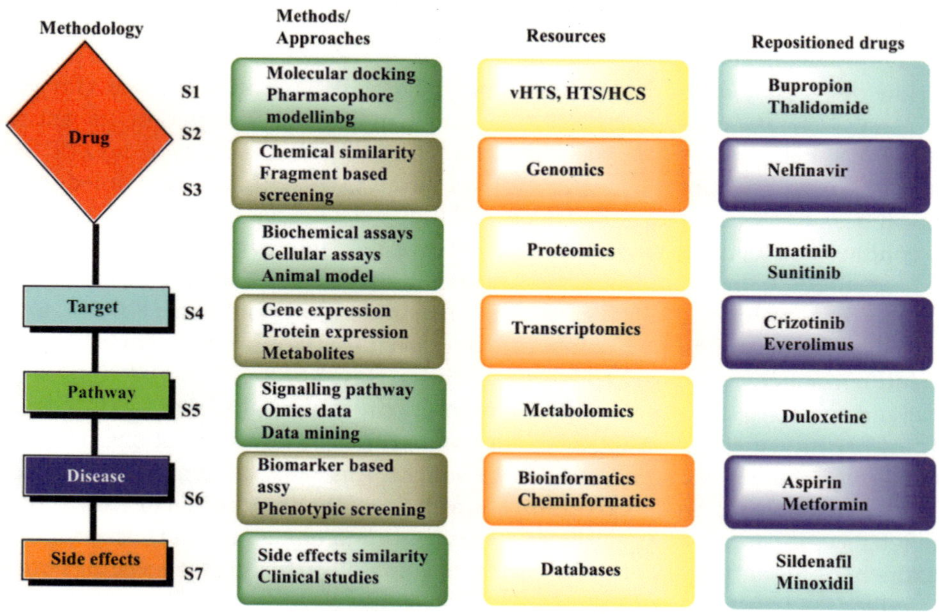

Figure 2.
Strategies of drug repositioning with examples.

4. Repurposed drugs

One alternate strategy to conventional drug discovery is drug repositioning. Due to rising market demand, many pharmaceutical companies are creating new medications or novel therapeutic applications for old, available pharmaceuticals through drug repositioning techniques in a shorter time and at a lower cost. The repositioning in a drug development program typically happens in two steps, which are as follows. The first step involves screening licensed medications *in silico* against a specific illness target. The second step involves further experimental investigation of the selected discovered molecules *in vitro* and *in vivo* in particular disease models of interest. The medication-chosen candidates move on to human clinical trials following the completion of fruitful preclinical research in the second stage of repositioning [18]. **Figure 2** delineates several potential strategies (with suitable examples) for drug repositioning.

Currently undergoing a clinical trial for the treatment of COVID-19 patients is colchicine, a well-known anti-inflammatory medication used to treat pericarditis and gout. This medication has been demonstrated to help avoid severe acute respiratory syndrome coronavirus-2 (SARS-CoV-2)-induced pneumonia from a massive cytokine storm. Worldwide research has also been done on the antiviral efficacy of an older antimalarial medication called chloroquine (as phosphate salt) against SARS-CoV-2 infection. Research indicates that chloroquine might help shield COVID-19 patients from coronavirus-induced pneumonia. According to recent reports from the US National Institutes of Health (NIH), a clinical trial combining azithromycin and hydroxychloroquine has already begun to treat COVID-19 patients. The FDA has approved both drugs in this combination—the antibacterial azithromycin and the antimalarial hydroxychloroquine. Currently, phase-2/phase-3 clinical studies are testing favipiravir, an antiviral medication used to treat influenza, on COVID-19 patients worldwide (China, Japan, the US, and India). Glenmark has initiated phase 3 favipiravir trials to treat COVID-19 patients in India. Remdesivir is an experimental antiretroviral drug being investigated in China, the US, the UK, and India to treat COVID-19 patients. Gilead Sciences Inc. originally developed it to treat Ebola, but it failed in a clinical trial. CSIR (Council of Scientific and Industrial Research) laboratories in India are conducting clinical trials on colchicine, remdesivir, and favipiravir. Several nations are now studying the use of lopinavir/ritonavir, a fixed-dose medication combination that was previously approved to treat HIV/AIDS under the brand name Kaletra, to treat COVID-19 patients. This combination of drugs was studied in conjunction with the influenza medication oseltamivir (Tamiflu) to treat SARS-CoV-2 infections in Thailand. Several locations worldwide are conducting a clinical trial of ivermectin, an anti-parasitic medication approved for use in treating worm infestations. This trial was started after Monash University in Melbourne, Australia, demonstrated the drug's effective treatment of SARS-CoV-2 infection *in vitro*. The clinical trial of tocilizumab, an IL-6 receptor antagonist (marketed under the brand name Actemra) used for the treatment of inflammatory illnesses such as rheumatoid arthritis, is also being conducted for the treatment of patients with COVID-19 [19, 20].

5. Recent advances in repurposed drugs

Recent advances in drug repurposing have highlighted the potential of existing drugs to treat a wide range of diseases beyond their original indications. By leveraging established safety profiles and accelerating clinical development, these repurposed drugs can provide new therapeutic options and address unmet medical needs.

5.1 COVID-19 pandemic

The majority of current antiviral medications, earlier developed or used as therapies for severe acute respiratory syndrome (SARS), HIV/AIDS, malaria, and Middle East respiratory syndrome (MERS), have been investigated as powerful COVID-19 treatments, with few transferring into clinical trials. Due to the rapid spread of COVID-19 and its high mortality, addressing the void for virus-specific drugs is urgent [21]. The coronavirus life cycle consists of various potentially targetable stages, as shown in **Figure 3**. The cellular receptor for SARS-CoV-2 is ACE2. Recombinant human ACE2 (rhACE2 or APN01) is currently under development for acute lung injury and pulmonary arterial hypertension. rhACE2 has been established to reduce viral entry into human-derived organoids [22]. Proteolysis of viral coat spike glycoprotein is required for viral entry into the cell, which TMPRSS2 can generally carry out. The ATMPRSS2 inhibitor Camostat was approved for treating chronic pancreatitis in Japan—camostat and nafamostat block SARS CoV-2 replication in ATMPRSS2-expressing human cells [23]. The clinical trials of these drugs to use in COVID-19 have already started in the Netherlands and Germany.

Before uncoating, the coronavirus uses the lysosomal pathway to enter the cells. Antimalarial quinine drugs such as Chloroquine (CQ) and Hydroxychloroquine (HCQ) inhibit this phenomenon in SARS CoV-2 replication. Azithromycin, a well-known broad-spectrum macrolide antibiotic, also proved to block autophagosome clearance [24]. RdRp carries both replication and transcription of the viral RNA,

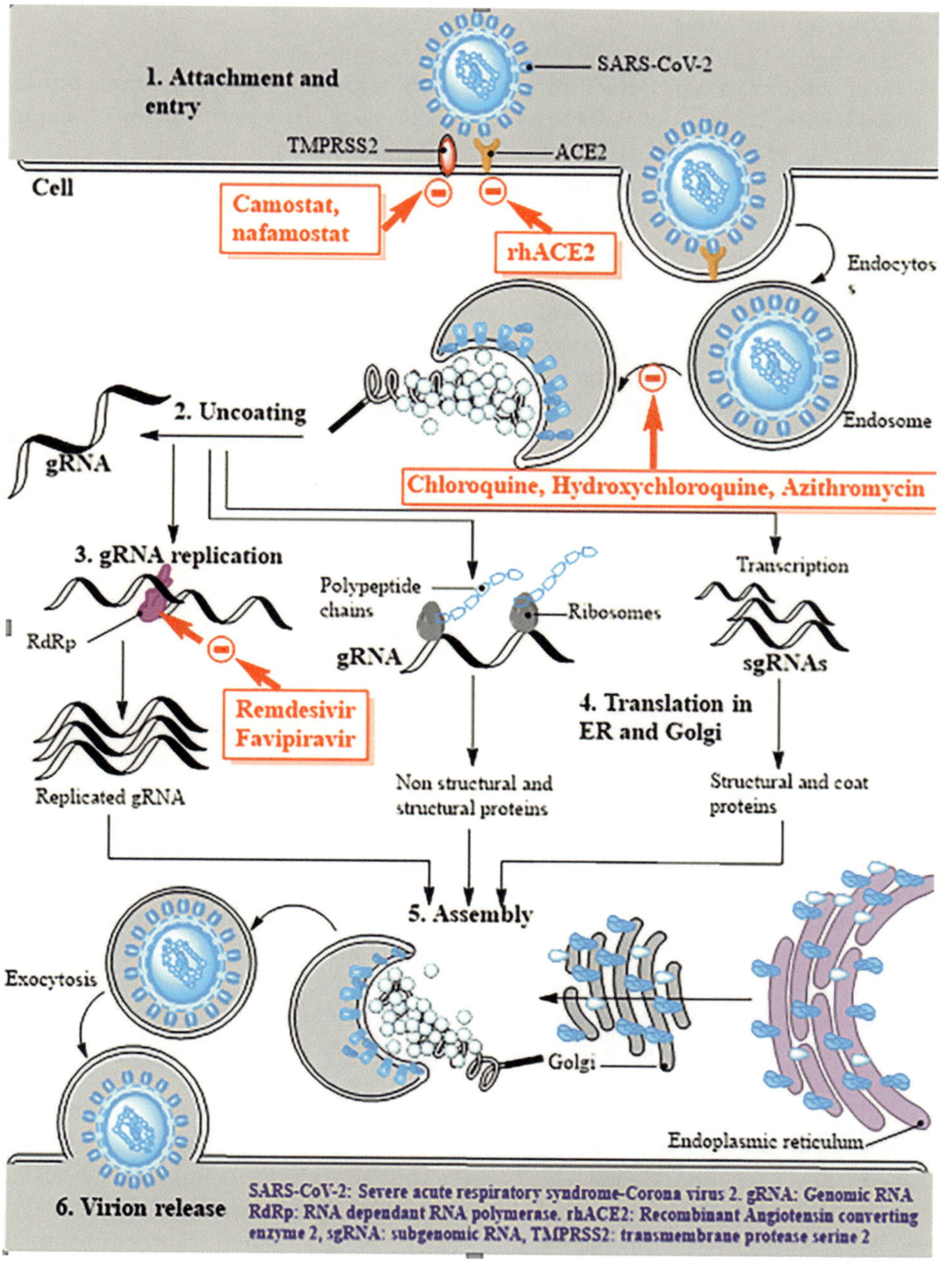

Figure 3.
Possible targets in corona virus life cycle; future repurposing of drugs could be focused on the above targets.

and its blockade can arrest the viral life cycle. RdRp is an acritical protein for many viruses, and several RdRp inhibitors are either approved or in clinical trials, including remdesivir and favipiravir [25]. Remdesivir, originally developed for Ebola, has been repurposed and approved for treating COVID-19, showing efficacy in reducing recovery time for hospitalized patients. Dexamethasone is a corticosteroid used for inflammatory conditions, and it has proven effective in reducing mortality in severely ill COVID-19 patients.

5.2 Anticancer therapies

Cancer stands as a top cause of mortality worldwide, having a remarkable burden on global health. Kirtonia et al. have reviewed the use of drug repurposing strategies in oncology. In recent years, Drug repurposing within the anticancer area has been boosted. Successful drugs like Busulfan and Chlorambucil were initially developed as Alkylating chemical warfare agents but were later found to be effective in treating leukemias. Thalidomide, a sedative drug, was repurposed as a leprotic myeloma drug. The 14 Hallmarks of Cancer must be well understood in order to repurpose the drugs for cancer treatment. There will be different mechanisms by which the repurposed Drug can affect the Tumor microenvironment (TME). Tumoroid models present a significant advancement in cancer drug screening due to their capacity to mimic the physical gene expressions and required characteristics and functionalities of their mother organs. SMAC mimetics like LCL161 have been evaluated for renal carcinoma, while YPN-005, a CDK7 inhibitor, has been systematically studied in the SCLC tumoroid system [26].

Phenotypic screening is a strategy that evaluates biology-associated (phenotypic) effects in the given models, such as animals, cells, or microorganisms, to help detect the drug targets; using this approach, some of the FDA-approved calcium channel blockers such as Amlodipine besylate, Felodipine, diclomanidipine, and cilidipine were observed to prevent cancer cell invasion by inhibition of filopodia formation [27].

Computational methodology has evolved as an essential tool in cancer drug repurposing methods. Evaluating cancer-specific pathway, inhibitor activity through computer-assisted drug repurposing approaches also denotes a sound process. Scientists can explore several databases of drug informatics, such as UCSC, Genbank, and many more, as represented in the table. Similarly, various network-based approaches can also be used to repurpose anticancer drugs [28].

Propranolol: A beta-blocker traditionally used for hypertension, propranolol is being explored for its anticancer properties, particularly in reducing the recurrence of breast cancer.

Itraconazole: An antifungal drug that has shown promise in inhibiting the Hedgehog signaling pathway, a target in certain cancers, including basal cell carcinoma (**Table 2**) [29].

Disulfiram, an alcohol antiabuse drug, was serendipitously identified for its ability to reduce metastasis of bone cancer cells. Disulfiram inhibits the glycolysis pathway of cancer cells in a copper dependent manner, thus altering the cellular metabolism. Oleanolic acid (OA, 3β-hydroxyolean-12-en-28-oic acid) is a terpenoid derived from plants and possesses antibacterial, antiparasitic, antidiabetic, and antitumor

Category	Name
Genome/target	UCSC, Genbank, Connectivity map, Ensembl, Gene ontology
Proteomics/ pathway	UniProt, UniGene, UniRef, KEGG, STRING, BiGRID, HAPPI, Reactome, The Human Protein Atlas
Disease data base	The cancer genome, Atlas, Cancer cell line encyclopedia, OMIM
Phenome	RepoDB, Clinical Trials, Drugs@FDA database, Drug bank

Table 2.
List of databases used in drug repurposing.

activities. OA was identified to inhibit the IL-1/NFκB/TET3 axis in tumor cells, resulting in nucleic acid hypomethylation and the suppression of PD-L1 by activating the T-cell defense mechanism. Tumor suppressor genes such as P53 are essential in regulating cancer progression. Some tumors can escape the P53 gene or turn off other tumor suppressors. In these cases, repurposed drugs may target such tumors and be beneficial. In inhibiting cholesterol synthesis, hyperlipidemic drug statins also block the synthesis of byproducts required for tumor cell growth. Simvastatin was observed to decrease the migration ability and invasive tendency of MDA-MB-231 breast cancer cells *in vitro* by increasing mutant P53 expression and decreasing the expression of stem cell marker CD44 (**Table 3** and **Figure 4**) [30, 31].

5.3 Neurodegenerative diseases

Drug repurposing for neurodegenerative diseases involves identifying existing medications, initially developed for other conditions, that can be used to treat diseases such as Alzheimer's, Parkinson's, and ALS. This approach leverages these drugs' known safety profiles and pharmacological data, potentially accelerating the development of effective treatments. Repurposing can significantly reduce the time and cost compared to traditional drug discovery, as these drugs have already undergone extensive testing for toxicity and side effects. By focusing on mechanisms such as neuroprotection, reducing neuroinflammation, and enhancing neuroregeneration, researchers hope to find new therapeutic uses for existing drugs, providing new hope for patients suffering from these debilitating diseases [32].

Repurposed drugs such as Dextromethorphan, commonly found in cough suppressants, are being studied for their neuroprotective and anti-inflammatory properties in conditions like ALS. Riluzole was initially approved for ALS but is being investigated for its neuroprotective effects in other neurodegenerative diseases

Drug	Methods	Disease
Metformin	DSPathNet	Breast, pancreas, and prostate cancers
	Mapping the proteomic profile on to SIGNOR data base	Breast cancer
	A structure-based method to identify proteome wide molecular weights of metformin	Various cancer types
	SMiR-NBI	Breast cancer
	SDTNBI	Various cancer types
Statins	Weighted gene co-expression network analysis and Cmap querying	Gastric cancer
	Cell cycle profiling	Various cancer types
	viper and PEANuT	Various cancer types
	MDP	Various cancer types
Protonpump inhibitor	Molecular docking	Pancreatic cancer and various types of cancers
Disulfiram	b-SDTNBI	Breast cancer

Table 3.
Drugs repurposed for cancer based on the network-based approaches.

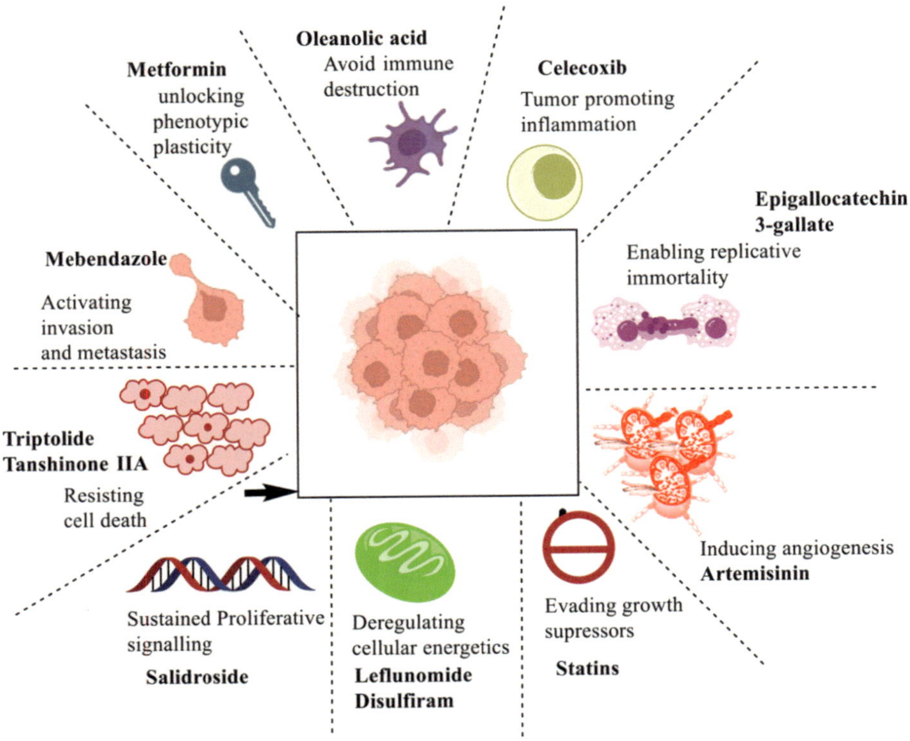

Figure 4.
Diverse cancer hallmarks targeted by repurposed non-oncology drugs.

like Alzheimer's and Huntington's disease [33]. Nilotinib, a leukemia drug, is being explored for its potential to clear toxic proteins and improve symptoms in Parkinson's and Alzheimer's diseases. Metformin is commonly used for diabetes; metformin is being studied for its potential to slow cognitive decline and improve outcomes in patients with Alzheimer's disease.

5.4 Antimicrobial resistance

Clofazimine: Initially developed for leprosy, clofazimine has shown effectiveness against multidrug-resistant tuberculosis (MDR-TB) and extensively drug-resistant TB (XDR-TB).

Bedaquiline: Originally developed for other bacterial infections, bedaquiline has been repurposed to treat MDR-TB, significantly improving treatment outcomes [34].

5.5 Host-directed therapies (HDTs)

Metformin: Beyond its antidiabetic effects, metformin is being explored for its ability to modulate the host immune response, potentially enhancing TB treatment.

Tyrosine Kinase Inhibitors: Drugs like imatinib, used in cancer treatment, are being investigated for their potential to boost immune responses against various infectious diseases [35].

5.6 Cardiovascular drugs in oncology

Statins: Commonly used to lower cholesterol, statins are being studied for their potential anticancer effects, particularly in reducing the risk of cancer recurrence and metastasis.

Aspirin: Long used for pain relief and cardiovascular protection, aspirin is now being investigated for its role in cancer prevention, especially colorectal cancer [36].

5.7 Anti-inflammatory drugs

Colchicine: Traditionally used for gout, colchicine is being repurposed for its anti-inflammatory effects in cardiovascular diseases, reducing the risk of heart attacks and strokes.

Naproxen: A nonsteroidal anti-inflammatory drug (NSAID), naproxen is under investigation for its potential to reduce the risk of colorectal cancer and Alzheimer's disease [37].

5.8 Psychiatric drugs

Ketamine: Originally an anesthetic, ketamine has shown rapid antidepressant effects in treatment-resistant depression, leading to the development of its derivative, esketamine, for depression treatment.

Lithium: Used for bipolar disorder, lithium is being explored for its neuroprotective properties in neurodegenerative diseases like Amyotropic lateral Sclerosis (ALS) and Alzheimer's disease [36].

6. Challenges

Repurposing drugs faces several challenges, including the need for rigorous scientific and clinical validation to demonstrate efficacy and safety for new indications. Regulatory hurdles require extensive documentation and new clinical data, complicating the approval process. Intellectual property issues, such as expired patents and difficulty securing new ones, can reduce financial incentives. Economic barriers deter investment, including high trial costs and uncertain market size. Designing appropriate clinical trials, addressing long-term safety concerns, and managing off-label use further complicate the process. Additionally, logistical challenges in manufacturing and distribution, alongside ethical considerations like equitable access and public perception, add to the complexity of repurposing drugs.

7. Future perspectives

7.1 Emerging areas for repurposing

Emerging areas for repurposing involve leveraging existing drugs, technologies, or knowledge in new and innovative ways to address unmet medical needs. This includes repurposing pharmaceuticals for different therapeutic indications, such as using cancer drugs to treat infectious diseases or exploring the use of established medical devices in novel applications like advanced robotics or telemedicine. Additionally, integrating artificial intelligence and machine learning to predict new uses for existing compounds is gaining traction, alongside the repurposing of data from clinical trials to identify new drug candidates. These approaches aim to accelerate drug development, reduce costs, and enhance the efficiency of medical research and treatment.

7.2 Innovative approaches

Innovative approaches in drug repurposing include leveraging computational methods such as artificial intelligence and machine learning to predict new therapeutic uses for existing drugs based on their molecular properties and biological effects. High-throughput screening of drug libraries against various disease models, combined with bioinformatics tools, helps identify potential repurposing candidates. Network pharmacology, which examines drug interactions and multiple targets, offers insights into new applications. Additionally, collaborative efforts between academia, industry, and regulatory agencies, along with real-world data from electronic health records and patient registries, enhance the identification and validation of repurposing opportunities, aiming to expedite the drug development process and reduce costs.

7.3 Challenges and solutions

Drug repurposing faces challenges such as intellectual property issues, regulatory hurdles, and limited financial incentives for pharmaceutical companies. Identifying appropriate candidates among the vast array of existing drugs requires extensive research and robust data analysis. Additionally, variations in drug formulations and dosages, initially designed for different conditions, can complicate repurposing efforts. Solutions to these challenges include:

- Fostering public-private partnerships to share data and resources
- Streamlining regulatory pathways to facilitate approvals
- Offering financial incentives or grants to encourage repurposing projects

Advances in computational tools and real-world data analytics also support the efficient identification and validation of potential repurposed drugs, addressing scientific and logistical obstacles.

7.4 Collaborative efforts

Collaborative efforts in drug repurposing involve partnerships between academic institutions, pharmaceutical companies, government agencies, and nonprofit organizations to share resources, data, and expertise. Initiatives like the National Institutes of Health's (NIH) National Center for Advancing Translational Sciences (NCATS) and the Open Innovation Drug Repurposing Initiative foster collaboration by providing platforms for sharing data and facilitating joint research projects. Public-private partnerships help overcome financial and logistical barriers by pooling resources and streamlining the drug repurposing process. These collaborations enhance the identification of promising drug candidates, accelerate clinical trials, and ultimately bring repurposed therapies to market more efficiently, benefiting patients with unmet medical needs.

8. Future research directions

Future research directions for drug repurposing are poised to harness advanced technologies and collaborative frameworks to uncover new therapeutic uses for existing drugs. One significant direction involves the integration of artificial intelligence and machine learning to analyze vast datasets, including genomic, proteomic, and clinical data, to predict potential drug–disease interactions. These computational approaches can identify previously overlooked relationships and streamline the selection of promising candidates for repurposing. Additionally, high-throughput screening techniques combined with CRISPR and other gene-editing technologies will enable more precise and efficient testing of drug effects on specific genetic targets, expanding the possibilities for personalized medicine.

Another critical area of future research is the development of comprehensive databases and platforms that facilitate sharing data and insights across the scientific community. Initiatives like the Illuminating the Druggable Genome (IDG) project aim to catalog and characterize understudied proteins, providing valuable information for repurposing efforts. Collaboration between academia, industry, and regulatory bodies will be crucial in establishing standardized protocols and regulatory frameworks to support drug repurposing. Furthermore, real-world evidence gathered from electronic health records, patient registries, and wearable devices will play an increasingly important role in identifying new applications for existing drugs and validating their efficacy in diverse patient populations. By leveraging these innovative approaches and fostering collaborative ecosystems, future research in drug repurposing can revolutionize healthcare and accelerate the discovery of novel treatments.

9. Critical views

Although drug repurposing is frequently praised for its ability to cut costs and development time, there are a number of serious disadvantages that need to be considered. Critics point out that repurposed medications still need to undergo costly and time-consuming clinical trials to demonstrate their usefulness for new applications, and they frequently face the same regulatory obstacles as new treatments despite the availability of safety data. Problems with intellectual property, like out-of-date patents and generic competition, can reduce business incentives and stifle innovation and investment. Repurposed medications may also have unanticipated adverse effects in novel settings, which would complicate their safety profile. Significant obstacles to their widespread adoption also include problems with off-label usage, logistical challenges in production and delivery, and assuring fair access.

10. Conclusion

In contemporary medicine, drug repurposing has shown great promise as a means of accelerating the release of medicines for a range of illnesses while cutting down on the expenses and duration of research and development. There have been significant advancements in medication repurposing in a variety of medical domains, including as neurodegenerative illnesses, cancer, infectious diseases, and more. Remdesivir and dexamethasone for COVID-19 are two well-known examples of how current medications can be quickly used to treat serious health emergencies. Progress in fields such as machine learning, computational biology, and high-throughput screening has also greatly improved the detection and verification of repurposed medication candidates.

But there are still a lot of obstacles to overcome. It is just as tricky as creating new medications requiring thorough clinical trials, regulatory approval, and rigorous scientific validation to ensure safety and efficacy for novel applications. The repurposing process is made more difficult by logistical difficulties, economic obstacles, and intellectual property concerns. There are significant obstacles in ensuring fair access and addressing ethical issues.

Drug repurposing has a bright future ahead of it thanks to continued research, creative thinking, and teamwork. AI and machine learning will remain essential in finding novel therapeutic applications for already approved medications. Utilizing genetic and phenotypic data, personalized medicine will assist in customizing repurposing medicines to each patient, increasing efficacy and reducing side effects. To ensure that innovations benefit a diverse range of patients worldwide, repurposing efforts must be advanced through public–private partnerships and global health initiatives.

In conclusion, even if the road to drug repurposing is complicated, it is essential to future medical research and development because of the possible time, money, and treatment choices. To solve current obstacles and realize the full promise of repurposed pharmaceuticals in enhancing global health outcomes, more innovation, cooperation, and funding in this area are necessary.

Conflict of interest

The authors declare that there is no conflict of interest.

Author details

Gatadi Srikanth[1*], Durga Prasad Beda[1] and Niggula Praveen Kumar[2]

1 School of Pharmacy, GITAM Deemed to be University, Hyderabad, India

2 Bharat Institute of Technology, Hyderabad, India

*Address all correspondence to: gatadi.srikanth8@gmail.com

References

[1] Cressey DJN. Traditional drug-discovery model ripe for reform. Nature. 2011;**471**(7336):17-18

[2] Jachak SM, Saklani A. Challenges and opportunities in drug discovery from plants. Current Science. 2007;**92**(9):1251-1257

[3] Khanna I. Drug discovery in pharmaceutical industry: Productivity challenges and trends. Drug Discovery Today. 2012;**17**(19-20):1088-1102

[4] Hua Y et al. Drug repositioning: Progress and challenges in drug discovery for various diseases. European Journal of Medicinal Chemistry. 2022;**234**:114239

[5] Oprea T, Mestres J. Drug repurposing: Far beyond new targets for old drugs. The AAPS Journal. 2012;**14**:759-763

[6] Pushpakom S et al. Drug repurposing: Progress, challenges and recommendations. Nature Reviews Drug discovery. 2019;**18**(1):41-58

[7] Gns HS et al. An update on drug repurposing: Re-written saga of the drug's fate. Biomedicine and Pharmacotherapy. 2019;**110**:700-716

[8] Phillips DJ. Pfizers expiring viagra patent adversely affects other drug makers too. Forbes. Jersey City, NJ: Forbes Media; 2013. Available from: https://www.forbes.com/sites/investor/2013/12/20/pfizers-expiring-viagra-patent-adversely-affects-other-drugmakers-too

[9] Ashburn TT, Tor KB. Drug repositioning: Identifying and developing new uses for existing drugs. Nature Reviews. Drug Discovery. 2004;**3**:673-683

[10] Urquhart L. Market watch; top drugs and companies by sales in 2017. Nature Reviews. Drug Discovery. 2018;**17**:232

[11] Sun W, Sanderson PE, Zheng W. Drug combination therapy increases successful drug repositioning. Drug Discovery Today. 2016;**21**(7):1189-1195

[12] Ma D-L, Chan DS-H, Leung C-H. Drug repositioning by structure-based virtual screening. Chemical Society Reviews. 2013;**42**(5):2130-2141

[13] Padhy B, Gupta Y. Drug repositioning: Re-investigating existing drugs for new therapeutic indications. Journal of Postgraduate Medicine. 2011;**57**(2):153

[14] Alshammari K, Taylor K, Siu LL. Efficacy considerations in phase I trials. In: Yap TA, Rodon J, Hong DS, editors. Phase I Oncology Drug Development. Cham: Springer; 2020. DOI: 10.1007/978-3-030-47682-3_10

[15] Paul D, Sanap G, Shenoy S, Kalyane D, Kalia K, Tekade RK. Artificial intelligence in drug discovery and development. Drug Discovery Today. 2021;**26**(1):80-93. DOI: 10.1016/j.drudis.2020.10.010

[16] Naylor S, Kauppi DM, Schonfeld JP. Therapeutic drug repurposing, repositioning and rescue part II: Business review. Drug Discovery World. 2015;**16**(2):57-72

[17] Parvathaneni V, Kulkarni NS, Muth A, Gupta V. Drug repurposing: A promising tool to accelerate the drug discovery process. Drug Discovery Today. 2019;**24**(10):2076-2085

[18] Liu Z, Fang H, Reagan K, Xu X, Mendrick DL, Slikker W, et al. In silico

drug repositioning – What we need to know. Drug Discovery Today. 2013;**18**(3-4):110-115

[19] March-Vila E, Pinzi L, Sturm N, Tinivella A, Engkvist O, Chen H, et al. On the integration of in silico drug design methods for drug repurposing. Frontiers in Pharmacology. 2017;**8**:1-12

[20] US FDA. FDA Cautions against Use of Hydroxychloroquine or Chloroquine for COVID-19 Outside of the Hospital Setting or a Clinical Trial Due to Risk of Heart Rhythm Problems. 2021. Available from: https://www.fda.gov/drugs/drug-safety-and-availability/fda-cautions-against-use-hydroxychloroquine-or-chloroquine-covid-19-outside-hospital-setting-or [Accessed: September 2, 2022]

[21] Kiplin Guy R, Dipaola RS, Romanelli F, Dutch RE. Rapid repurposing of drugs for covid-19. Science. 2020;**368**(6493):829-830

[22] Lan J, Ge J, Yu J, et al. Structure of the SARS-CoV-2 spike receptor-binding domain bound to the ACE2 receptor. Nature. 2020;**581**:215-220

[23] Hoffmann M, Weber HK, Schroeder S, Kruger N, Herrler T, Erichsen S, et al. SARS-CoV-2 cell entry depends on ACE2 and TMPRSS2 and is blocked by a clinically proven protease inhibitor. Cell. 2020;**181**(2):271-280

[24] Mauthe M, Orhon I, Rocchi C, Zhou X, Luhr M, Hijlkema KJ, et al. Chloroquine inhibits autophagic flux by decreasing autophagosome-lysosome fusion. Autophagy. 2018;**14**(8):1435-1455

[25] Arrowsmith J. Phase III and submission failures: 2007-2010. Nature Reviews. Drug Discovery. 2011;**10**(2):87

[26] Choi YJ et al. Discovery of a novel CDK7 inhibitor YPN-005 in small cell lung cancer. European Journal of Pharmacology. 2021;**907**:174298

[27] Jacquemet G et al. L-type calcium channels regulate filopodia stability and cancer cell invasion downstream of integrin signalling. Nature Communications. 2016;**7**:13297

[28] Ahmed F, Samantasinghar A, Ali W. et al. Network-based drug repurposing identifies small molecule drugs as immune checkpoint inhibitors for endometrial cancer. Molecular Diversity. 2024. DOI: 10.1007/s11030-023-10784-7

[29] Chong RX et al. Repurposing itraconazole as an anticancer agent. Oncology Letters. 2017;**14**:2582-2594

[30] Andal CC, Ghosh-Choudhury N, Yoneda T, Choudhury GG, Ghosh Choudhury N. Simvastatin prevents skeletal metastasis of breast cancer by an antagonistic interplay between p53 and CD44. The Journal of Biological Chemistry. 2011;**286**:11314-11327

[31] Shah S, Dooms MM, Amaral-Garcia S, Igoillo-Esteve M. Current drug repurposing strategies for rare neurodegenerative disorders. Frontiers in Pharmacology. 2021;**12**:56-63

[32] Kho S, Seung KJ, Huerga H, Bastard M, Khan PY, Mitnick CD, et al. Sputum culture reversion in longer treatments with bedaquiline, delamanid, and repurposed drugs for drug-resistant tuberculosis. Nature Communications. 2024;**15**(1):53-64

[33] Kakoti BB, Bezbaruah R, Ahmed N. Therapeutic drug repositioning with special emphasis on neurodegenerative diseases: Threats and issues. Frontiers in Pharmacology. 2022;**13**:1007315. DOI: 10.3389/fphar.2022.1007315

[34] Druker BJ, Lydon NB. Lessons learned from the development of an abl tyrosine kinase inhibitor for chronic myelogenous leukemia. Journal of Clinical Investigation. 2000;**105**(1):3-7

[35] Antithrombotic Trialists' Collaboration. Collaborative meta-analysis of randomised trials of antiplatelet therapy for prevention of death, myocardial infarction, and stroke in high risk patients. BMJ. 2002;**324**(7329):71-86

[36] Martin BK, Szekely C, Brandt J, et al. Cognitive function over time in the Alzheimer's disease anti-inflammatory prevention trial (ADAPT): Results of a randomized, controlled trial of naproxen and celecoxib. Archives of Neurology. 2008;**65**(7):896-905

[37] MacDonald A, Briggs K. Lithium therapy and its potential role in Alzheimer's disease. Current Alzheimer Research. 2015;**12**(8):849-853

Chapter 3

Drug Repositioning in the AI-Driven Era: Data, Approaches, and Challenges

Jing Wang, Siming Kong, Xiaochen Bo, Yunfang Wang, Song He and Hui Bai

Abstract

The advent of artificial intelligence (AI) has revolutionized drug repositioning, transforming it into an indispensable strategy for accelerating drug discovery. This chapter offers an in-depth exploration of the multifaceted landscape of drug repositioning in the AI era, emphasizing the profound influence of AI on this domain and providing a roadmap for future research. Beginning with a brief summary of the data that form the bedrock of this field, biomedical databases encompassing drugs, diseases, molecular targets, and clinical data are introduced in detail. Then the experimental and computational approaches that underpin drug repositioning are further dissected, ranging from binding assays or phenotypic screening to the multi-omics methodologies and in silico technologies, with emphasis on AI-driven methods. Subsequently, successful drug repositioning cases across diverse diseases are highlighted. Finally, the importance of fully leveraging AI to address challenges in drug repositioning is underscored.

Keywords: drug repositioning, artificial intelligence, biomedical databases, machine learning, phenotypic screening, computational modeling

1. Introduction

Drug repositioning, also known as drug repurposing, is the process of discovering new indications for existing drugs [1]. This approach leverages the extensive safety and efficacy data already available for approved drugs or compounds in development, thereby accelerating the drug development process and reducing its associated costs and risks. Traditionally, this process has been rooted in serendipitous clinical observations, such as the repositioning of amantadine, which was unexpectedly found during a patient's case observation in 1968 [2]. Such methods, while occasionally fruitful, were often inefficient and relied on chance findings.

The advent of computational methods has significantly accelerated drug repositioning research. Techniques like molecular docking [3–5] and molecular dynamics simulations [6–8] empowered researchers to predict and analyze the interactions between drugs and their targets with greater precision and speed. The omics-based methods combine various types of omics data to reveal the underlying mechanisms of diseases, discover potential therapeutic targets, and facilitate the drug repositioning process [9–13]. Network-based methods utilize the topology of biological networks to uncover possible novel applications for current medications [14–16]. These approaches allowed for a more systematic exploration of the potential of existing drugs beyond their original indications.

While the aforementioned computational methods have significantly accelerated drug repositioning research, they encounter inherent limitations when confronted with the multimodal and vast biomedical datasets. Also, they may not fully address the complexity and variety of tasks involved in drug repositioning. In the era of AI-driven techniques like ChatGPT and AlphaFold [17–19], there is an increasing interest in applying AI techniques for drug repositioning. The integration of AI technologies with biomedical data has enabled researchers to uncover complex patterns and relationships that were previously undetectable within biological data, leading to a paradigm shift in drug discovery and development. For instance, text mining significantly enhances the efficiency of information retrieval, facilitating the integration of information for drug repositioning [20]. Moreover, the primary AI method utilized for drug repositioning, machine learning, is widely applied for multiple tasks, such as drug-target relationship prediction [21–23], drug response prediction [24–26], and drug combination prediction [27–29]. These AI technologies have accelerated the pace of drug repositioning.

This chapter, "Drug repositioning in the AI-driven era: data, approaches, and challenges," aims to provide a comprehensive overview of the current state of drug repositioning, with a focus on the role of AI in this domain. It starts with the various databases that form the backbone of drug repositioning efforts, exploring how they contribute distinct yet complementary information to the field. Next, this chapter explores the multifaceted computational methods for drug repositioning. Structure-based methods, omics-based methods, network-based methods, and machine learning-based methods are discussed, with a focus on machine learning-based methods. Moreover, this chapter also review the role of binding assays and phenotypic screening for drug repositioning. Finally, the chapter summarizes the progress achieved and the challenges faced for drug repositioning, reflecting on the journey so far and the path forward.

2. Databases supporting drug repositioning

Drug repositioning is a multifaceted process that relies heavily on a variety of specialized databases. Each type of database contributes distinct yet complementary information, forming a collective knowledge base that accelerates the discovery of new therapeutic applications for existing drugs. This section summarizes databases supporting drug repositioning.

2.1 Drug related databases

Drug related databases collect a rich source of information about drugs. They compile a wealth of data encompassing drug structures, properties, and their relationship to various targets or diseases. Take DrugBank [30], for example; it is celebrated for its exhaustive data of drug-related information, including but not limited to molecular structure, drug target, ATC code, and indications. Molecular structure can be used in structure-based drug repositioning methods, which apply docking or molecular dynamics simulation to screen drug targets to identify novel indications. Also, molecular structure and other drug property information can be used in network-based methods or used as input features for machine learning methods. PubChem [31], with its extensive collection of chemical substances, supports the exploration of chemical properties (not only drugs) and bioactivities. These databases serve as a foundation for drug repositioning by offering insights into drug characteristics and potential interactions with biological systems.

In addition to individual drug information databases, there are also databases that collect data on drug combinations, such as DrugComb [32]; these databases provide a data foundation for the drug repositioning of drug combinations. More databases are provided in **Table 1**.

Category	Databases	Description	Website
Drug	DrugBank [30]	Molecular structure; drug target; ATC code; indications; side effect; drug-drug interaction	https://go.drugbank.com/
	PubChem [31]	Molecular structure; ATC code; indications; side effect;	https://pubchem.ncbi.nlm.nih.gov/
	CHEMBL [33]	Molecular structure; drug target; Indications;	https://www.ebi.ac.uk/chembl/
	Sider [34]	Indications; side effect	http://sideeffects.embl.de/
	DrugComb [32]	Drug combinations	https://drugcomb.fimm.fi/
	DrugCombDB [35]	Drug combinations	http://drugcombdb.denglab.org/
Gene/protein	Universal Protein (UniProt) [36]	Protein sequence; gene terms; protein-protein interactions; 3D structures of proteins	https://www.uniprot.org/
	Protein Data Bank (PDB) [37]	3D structures of proteins; protein sequence	http://www.rcsb.org
	Gene Ontology(GO) [38]	Functions of gene and gene products	https://www.geneontology.org/
	Kyoto Encyclopedia of Genes and Genomes (KEGG) [39]	Pathway	http://www.kegg.jp/
	Biological General Repository for Interaction Datasets (BioGrid) [40]	Protein-protein interactions; gene-gene interactions	https://thebiogrid.org
	Human Protein Reference Database (HPRD) [41]	Protein sequence; protein-protein interactions	http://www.hprd.org/
	Search Tool for the Retrieval of Interaction Gene/Proteins (STRING) [42]	Protein-protein interactions	https://cn.string-db.org/

Category	Databases	Description	Website
Disease	Online Mendelian Inheritance in Man (OMIM)	Human genes and genetic phenotypes	http://omim.org
	Disease Gene Network (DisGeNET) [43]	Associated genes	https://disease-ontology.org/
	Disease ontology [44]	Disease phenotypes; disease terms	http://www.disease-ontology.org
	The human phenotype ontology(HPO) [45]	Disease phenotypes; disease terms	https://hpo.jax.org/
Clinical data	ClinicalTrials	Contains clinical studies, adverse effects; disease indications	https://clinicaltrials.gov/
	Drugs@FDA	FDA approved drugs and their dosage information	https://www.accessdata.fda.gov/scripts/cder/daf/
	UK Biobank	Genome, transcriptome proteome, metabolome, and phenome of UK participants	https://www.ukbiobank.ac.uk/
Drug omics	The Connectivity Map(cMap) [46]	Perturbed expression profiles to chemical or genetic perturbation	https://clue.io
	Genomics of drug sensitivity in cancer (GDSC) [47]	Somatic mutations, copy number variations, DNA methylation, and gene expression profiles of cancer cell lines; cancer cell lines sensitivity to compounds	http://www.cancerrxgene.org/

Table 1.
Summary of the databases supporting drug repositioning.

2.2 Gene/protein related databases

Gene and protein-related databases provide a foundation for understanding the molecular targets of drugs. These databases include sequences and 3D structure properties (e.g., UniProt [36], PDB [37]), functional properties (e.g., GO [38], KEGG [39]), and topological properties in protein-protein interactions (PPI) (e.g., STRING [42], HPRD [41], BioGrid [40]), as shown in **Table 1**. Protein 3D structure information supports structure-based drug repositioning methods to explore the affinity between drugs and targets. Sequences and 3D structure, functional and topological properties are generally used in drug-target prediction based on network or machine learning methods. Consequently, these databases are vital for identifying drug targets and facilitating drug repositioning efforts.

2.3 Disease related databases

Disease-related databases are pivotal for linking drugs to potential new indications. The genetic information (e.g., OMIM, DisGeNET [43]) of disease can enable researchers to understand diseases at the molecular level, which is usually applied in Mendelian randomization or network-based methods. The disease terms (e.g., Disease ontology [44], HPO [45]) usually present some key information about the phenotype of a disease. This information is invaluable for the process of drug repositioning through disease similarity construction in machine learning or network-based methods. By integrating these diverse data sources, researchers can identify previously unrecognized connections between drugs and diseases, potentially leading to the discovery of novel treatments.

2.4 Clinical data related databases

Clinical databases are instrumental in the drug repositioning process by providing a rich source of clinical information that can be leveraged to identify new therapeutic opportunities for existing medications. Taking UK Biobank as an example, this large-scale biomedical database contains gene expression data derived from various tissues, including blood, adipose tissue and brain samples; measurements of various proteins in biological samples; and metabolomic profiling that captures the small molecules present in biological samples, such as blood or urine. These data are usually used in Mendelian randomization, omics-based methods or retrospective case-control pharmacoepidemiologic analyses [48] for drug repositioning.

2.5 Drug omics databases

Drug omics databases contain omics data of cell lines. GDSC database [47], for instance, contains somatic mutations, copy number variations, DNA methylation, and gene expression profiles of numerous cancer cell lines, as well as drug response data, which can be used in drug response prediction. CMap [46] offers a comprehensive repository of gene expression profiles obtained from the systematic perturbations to cell lines, including perturbations caused by small molecules and genes. This database facilitates the establishment of connections between diseases, genes, and pharmaceuticals by deciphering the molecular signatures induced by small molecules or genes [46, 49]. In drug repositioning field, cMap data are widely used in signature-based methods or used as input features of the drugs in machine learning methods.

3. Computational modeling for drug repositioning

Computational modeling for drug repositioning encompasses a wide array of methods, each with its unique strengths and applications. In this section, we delve into the specifics of these computational approaches, exploring their methodologies and applications in the context of drug repositioning. These methods include structure-based methods, omics-based methods, network-based methods, and machine learning methods (**Figure 1**). The specific comparisons of these computational methods are presented in **Table 2**; the databases involved in specific representative works are summarized in **Table 3**.

3.1 Structure-based methods

Structure-based methods focus on exploring the potential interactions between drugs and molecular targets, aiming to uncover novel applications for existing drugs. The two common structure-based drug repositioning methods are molecular docking and molecular dynamic.

Molecular docking is a computational strategy based on the structure to predict the binding site complementarity between the ligand (e.g., a drug) and the target (e.g., a receptor) [5]. Docking plays a pivotal role in drug repositioning by enabling the screening of drug libraries against a specific disease target or exploring multiple

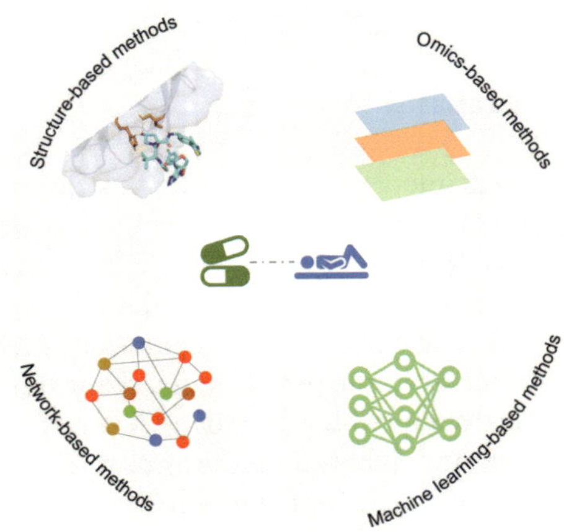

Figure 1.
Common computational methods for drug repositioning.

Methods	Description	Advantages	Disadvantages
Structure-based methods	Investigates structural complementarity between drugs and targets to predict binding affinity	Provides molecular insights into how drugs work	Dependency on structural information; not applicable to multi-target diseases; only applicable to the prediction of drug-target relationship
Omics-based methods	Integrates multi-omics data to understand the mechanism disease or drug	More comprehensive view of the underlying mechanisms; enable personalized medicine	Dependency on the quality and availability of omics data; data integration challenges
Network-based methods	Leverages the topology of biological networks to identify potential new uses for existing drugs	A more comprehensive understanding of the interaction of drugs, targets or other biological entities	Lack of specificity; network data is incomplete and contains a lot of noises
Machine learning-based methods	Applies algorithms to fit patterns behind the data to make predictions for various tasks	Uncovers hidden patterns from the known data; suitable for multiple tasks in the field of drug repositioning; adapts to large datasets	Sensitive to data quality; May lack interpretability

Table 2.
Summary of computational methods for drug repositioning.

targets against one drug (typically referred to as reverse molecular docking) [54]. Currently, the availability of diverse software like AutoDock [55], GOLD [56], FlexX [57], Surflex [58], and GLIDE [59] aids researchers in enhancing docking's accuracy and efficiency. However, several challenges accompany the use of docking for drug repositioning. One significant hurdle is the lack of available 3D structures for some protein targets, particularly membrane proteins like G Protein-Coupled Receptors [3]. Additionally, there is a scarcity of well-curated databases that offer accurate structural information for macromolecular targets [60]. Furthermore, the predictive accuracy of docking algorithms regarding binding affinity has been questioned.

Methods	Databases	Data description
Structure-based methods [8]	PDB [37]	69,843 Structures of human sequences
	PubChem [31]	118,564,728 Unique chemical structures
Omics-based methods [50, 51]	UK Biobank	Whole genome sequencing for all 500,000 participants
	cMap [46]	Gene expression profiles under 19,000 small molecules perturbations
Network-based methods [16]	SM2miR [52]	Experimentally validated small molecules' effects on miRNA expression. Number of miRNAs: 1658 Number of small molecules: 255 Number of entries: 4989
	PubChem [31]	118,564,728 Unique chemical structures
Machine learning-based methods [21, 25, 27]	Novartis' internal in silico activity dataset	5.5 million compounds (Novartis in-house resources)
	cMap [46]	Gene expression profiles under 5000 genetic perturbations
	GO [38]	42,093 GO terms 1,537,645 gene products
	Cancer Cell Line Encyclopedia (CCLE) [53]	Structural variants for 329 cell lines
	GDSC [47]	969 Cell lines 297 Compounds 243,466 IC50s
	PubChem [31]	118,564,728 Unique chemical structures
	DrugComb [32]	739,964 Drug combinations

Table 3.
Summary of databases involved in some representative works.

While improvements are ongoing, variations exist between different software packages, and certain limitations, such as predicting binding modes and entropic effects, persist [54, 61, 62].

Molecular dynamics (MD) simulation is a computational method that provides a detailed description of the behavior and motion of atoms and molecules over time [8]. By employing mathematical models known as force fields, molecular dynamics simulations explore the potential energy surface of a system, offering insights into its dynamic properties, including conformational transitions, structural changes, and interactions with other molecules or environments [6]. These simulations are instrumental in studying a variety of phenomena such as protein folding and drug binding [7]. When integrated with molecular docking, MD simulations can significantly enhance the reliability of docking results [63]. Docking identifies potential drug-target interactions, while MD simulations provide a deeper understanding of the dynamic behavior of these interactions, accounting for factors such as entropic effects and conformational changes that may not be fully captured by docking alone. This combination of techniques allows for a more comprehensive evaluation of drug-target binding. Sadeghi et al. [8] applied molecular docking to screen DrugBank-approved compounds for potential interactions with α-glucosidase, a key enzyme in diabetes treatment. Then they used molecular dynamics simulations to verify the stability of the most promising compound-docked complexes. The combined use of these computational techniques identified Forodesine as a competitive inhibitor with a low half maximum inhibitory concentration (IC_{50}) value, suggesting its potential as a novel therapeutic agent for diabetes through α-glucosidase inhibition.

3.2 Omics-based methods

Omics-based methods apply single or multi-omics data to understand disease mechanisms, identify new drug targets, and guide the repositioning process [11]. In general, these methods apply statistics-based methods to apply genome-wide association study (GWAS) [64], transcriptome-wide association study (TWAS) [10], or proteome-wide association study (PWAS) [9], so as to identify novel drug targets for specific diseases. For instance, Chen et al. [65] developed TESLA, an approach integrating an expression quantitative trait locus dataset with multi-ancestry GWAS. Applied to tobacco use phenotypes, they identify 273 new genes and highlight potential drugs for nicotine addiction treatment, including dextromethorphan and galantamine.

In the subsequent sections, we will explore two additional omics technologies that are widely applied in drug repurposing: Mendelian randomization and signature-based methods.

3.2.1 Mendelian randomization

Mendelian randomization (MR) employs genetic variants as instrumental variables to infer causal relationships between drug targets and outcomes [11], offering a robust approach to drug repositioning by mitigating confounding factors and reverse causation inherent in observational data. Applied 2-sample Mendelian randomization study (Collecting exposure and outcome data from two separate, non-overlapping populations), Tang et al. [50] identifies an association between genetic variations in sulfonylurea antidiabetic drug targets and a reduced risk of Alzheimer's disease, highlighting the sulfonylurea class as a potential therapeutic area for further exploration in Alzheimer's prevention and treatment.

MR is not influenced by confounding factors, providing a clear line of sight to causal relationships between drug targets and diseases based on the genome data. However, its applicability is restricted to drugs with strong genetic predictors, and it may fall short for drugs where the genetic determinants are weak or complex.

3.2.2 Signature-based methods

A gene signature refers to the distinctive pattern of expression profile in cells that is associated with specific normal or disease processes, as well as responses to drug treatment [66]. CMap is a reference database that contains gene expression profiles resulting from systematic perturbation treatments of compounds or genes, which provides valuable gene signature data. Signature-based drug repositioning methods involve two primary strategies: drug-disease approaches and drug-drug approaches [54].

Drug-disease approaches are based on the presumption that the drug capable of restoring disease-induced gene signatures back to their normal state could potentially serve as a therapeutic candidate for treating the disease [67]. Many studies follow this principle, leveraging drug perturbation expression profiles from CMap to discover repositioned drugs for particular diseases. The key of these studies lies in acquiring disease-related expression profiles and establishing computational methods to match disease expression profiles with drug expression profiles, with the aim of repositioning therapeutic drugs for specific diseases. For instance, in their search for novel treatments for Human adenoviruses (HAdV) infections, Wang *et al.* [51] measured the transcriptome data of HAdV-infected human lung epithelial cells. Then they employed the Gene Set Enrichment Analysis (GSEA) method to match the disease expression profile and drug perturbation expression profiles from CMap. Through this process, they identified the anti-diabetic drug rosiglitazone as a potential treatment for HAdV infections, with experimental results confirming its efficacy both *in vitro* and *in vivo*.

Drug-drug approaches are premised on the idea that if two drugs share a common transcriptomic signature, they may also possess similar therapeutic applications, irrespective of the similarities or differences in their chemical structures [12, 68]. The key to these approaches lies in computing drug-drug similarity, often in combination with other computational methods such as network-based methods. Iorio et al. leveraged gene signature data to construct drug similarity networks, enabling the repositioning of fasudil, a Rho-kinase (ROCK) inhibitor to be an enhancer of cellular autophagy, with therapeutic effects in several neurodegenerative conditions [13, 68].

3.3 Network-based methods

In biological networks, each node represents an interacting entity (drug, disease, gene, non-coding RNA, protein, or other biomedical entities), while the edges represent their various interactions or relationships, such as functional similarities or regulatory relationship [69]. Network-based methods leverage the topology of biological networks to identify potential new uses for existing drugs. For instance, Zhou et al. [16] construct drug-drug interaction network based on curated drug-miRNA associations and found topology densely connected drugs tend to share similar therapeutic effects in the drug-drug interaction network. Additionally, network-based methods frequently employ graph mining algorithms like random walk, path search and network propagation to uncover potential connections between drug and disease that were previously unlinked within a heterogeneous network [15]. Wang et al. [14] proposed a novel drug repositioning strategy termed “Drug Repositioning-based on Individual Bi-random Walks” (DR-IBRW). This approach overcomes the limitations of existing random walk-based methods that overlook varying node contributions in information transfer and typically adopt a fixed walk-length for all nodes. DR-IBRW uses disease and drug information to construct disease-disease and drug-drug similarity networks, calculates an individual walk-length for each node based on the topology of drug-disease network. It then performs quantified bi-random walks to account for structural differences among these networks, varying node contributions, and identify new drug-disease associations.

Network-based methods capitalize on topology of biological networks and provide a broader understanding of the interactions among drugs, targets, and other biological entities. However, the lack of specificity and the prevalence of incomplete and noisy data in biological networks can limit the accuracy and reliability of predictions made by these methods.

3.4 Machine learning-based methods

In the field of drug repositioning, from target identification to drug-target prediction, machine learning methods play a crucial role with its ability to recognize complex patterns behind large datasets. Traditional machine learning methods, such as support vector machine and random forest, rely on handcrafted features. Furthermore, deep learning methods, including convolutional neural network, recurrent neural network, and graph neural network (GNN) can automatically extract complex features from unstructured data, such as molecular structures and genomic sequences.

One of the critical tasks in drug repositioning is the prediction of drug-target relationship, which is essential for identifying potential novel uses for marketed or failed drugs. In addition to drug-target prediction, machine learning techniques are also employed in other tasks such as drug response prediction, drug property prediction, and exploration of drug-disease associations. This section will delve into the application of machine learning in drug repositioning, focusing on drug-target prediction and other related tasks.

3.4.1 Drug-target relationship prediction

Drug-target relationship prediction by machine learning models can help us to find potential novel uses of exited drugs. The primary task of these models is to predict whether a drug can bind to a specific target. For instance, DeepConv-DTI [23] utilizes convolutional neural networks to predict the likelihood of an interaction between a drug and a target based on drug fingerprint and protein sequence data. This work performed convolution on different lengths of amino acid subsequences to capture local residue patterns of target. GNN excel at capturing complex patterns on graph. Shao et al. [22] constructed a heterogeneous graph from drug and target similarity matrices alongside drug-target interaction (DTI) data. The proposed model, DTI-HETA, integrates this graph with an attention mechanism for precise DTI prediction. In addition to algorithm design, information effectiveness behind the input features is also crucial for the prediction task. Inspired by the word2vec technique in natural language processing, Chen et al. [21] developed the Functional Representation of Gene Signatures (FRoGS) model, which encapsulates gene signatures in terms of their biological functions. FRoGS has been proven to be superior in predicting drug-target interactions compared to methods that solely rely on gene identity.

Machine learning models are also applied in other drug-target prediction related tasks, such as binding affinities or binding site prediction. Li et al. have developed an innovative model known as Co-VAE (co-regularized variational autoencoders), which uses the structure of drugs and the sequence of targets to predict binding affinities, also aiding in discovering drugs that hit similar targets [70]. Pan et al. [71] proposed BindingSiteDTI, which is a deep learning model that enhances drug-target interaction prediction by intelligently scaling features to achieve binding site prediction. More recently, cutting-edge advancements like AlphaFold3 [18], with its advanced diffusion-based framework, have pushed the boundaries further by predicting complex structures involving proteins and small molecules. These models provide deeper insights into drug-target interactions, which is crucial for understanding their therapeutic potential.

3.4.2 Drug-disease association prediction

Drug–disease association prediction provides direct information for drug repositioning, identifying new therapeutic potentials for specific diseases. This method leverages comprehensive data, such as disease-disease associations or drug-drug associations to predict novel drug-disease associations. One of the representative works is HNet-DNN model [72], which extracted topological features within drug-disease heterogeneous networks to train a deep neural network to predict novel drug-disease associations. And more recently, GNN demonstrated excellent performance on graph-based tasks, Meng et al. [73] developed DRAGNN, a novel graph neural network model that dynamically prioritizes information from heterogeneous drug and disease nodes using a graph attention mechanism, while strategically omitting self-node aggregation to preserve valuable network embeddings. The model simplifies neighbor information aggregation through average pooling and employs a multi-layer perceptron for drug-disease association prediction, demonstrating robust effectiveness.

3.4.3 Drug response prediction

Drug response prediction plays a pivotal role in the realm of drug repositioning by providing insights into how different cell lines or preclinical models may respond to a particular medication [24–26, 74–76]. For cellular response prediction, the majority of studies [24–26, 75] harness the omics feature of cell lines in conjunction with the fingerprint or molecular graph of the drugs to achieve novel drug-cell line response prediction. A case in point is the model proposed by Kuenzi et al., known as DrugCell, which is an interpretable deep neural network embedded with gene-related knowledge. This model utilizes input mutation data of cell lines combined with drug fingerprints to predict drug response to cell lines. For drug response prediction for preclinical models, studies [74, 76] usually apply transfer learning methods to address the problem of small preclinical samples.

3.4.4 Drug property prediction

Drug property prediction is a key field in drug repositioning, especially in predicting the therapeutic properties of drugs. The Anatomical Therapeutic Chemical (ATC) classification system is an internationally recognized drug categorization framework maintained by the World Health Organization's (WHO) collaborating centers. It classifies medications based on the anatomical site of action, therapeutic use, and chemical characteristics, facilitating standardized and comparative drug usage. Machine learning methods have emerged as a powerful tool in the prediction of ATC classifications for drugs. For instance, Xie et al. [77] introduced a novel domain-adversarial multi-task framework for predicting ATC classifications of drugs, with the innovation of using an adversarial strategy and multi-task framework to model the nonlinear dependencies among heterogeneous data to enhance the accuracy of the prediction. The model has effectively facilitated the repositioning of FDA-approved drugs by identifying their potential for new therapeutic applications, as evidenced by the successful prediction and retrospective analysis of drugs like mecamylamine for anti-depressant and anti-addictive indications.

Besides, accurate prediction of drug properties, such as absorption, distribution, metabolism, excretion and toxicity (ADMET), is essential for assessing the druggability of compounds. One of the representative works, ADMETlab [78–80], is an integrated online webserver that offers precise predictions for ADMET characteristics. Utilizing multi-task deep message passing neural networks (DMPNN), it provides a robust, high-throughput platform for analyzing a comprehensive suite of ADMET properties. ADMETlab 3.0 is readily accessible to the public without requiring registration and can be found at: https://admetlab3.scbdd.com.

3.4.5 Drug combination prediction

Given the limitations of single-drug potency that restrict the clinical applicability in drug repositioning, the vast potential of combination therapy emerges as a promising alternative, offering a broader array of options to enhance the success of drug repositioning [29]. Machine learning methods demonstrate significant efficacy in predicting drug combinations, typically framing the task as either a multi-class classification or a regression problem. Specifically, the combined effects of drugs are categorized into synergistic, additive, and antagonistic based on established definitions [28]. Yet, the predominant focus in classification studies is the binary division into synergistic and non-synergistic categories, which poses an imbalanced classification challenge. Wu et al. [27] proposed ForSyn, an advanced deep forest-based approach, to effectively address the issue of imbalanced classification on small-scale, high-dimensional datasets. Additionally, interpretability is also crucial for drug combination prediction. Additionally, interpretability is also crucial for drug combination prediction. By employing feature attribution techniques, Janizek et al. [81] demonstrate that the explanations can be enhanced through the use of multiple interpretable machine-learning models. Combined biological process network with deep neural network, Wang et al. developed an interpretable framework for designing synthetic lethality-based combination therapies.

4. Experimental approaches for drug repositioning

This section introduces the main experimental approaches for drug repositioning, including binding assays and phenotypic screening. Binding assays facilitate drug repositioning by revealing new drug-target interactions, which is advantageous for deciphering drug mechanisms. However, this approach may not be ideal for drugs exerting their effects through interactions with multiple targets simultaneously. Phenotypic screening, which assesses the effects of drugs on observable traits in biological systems, allows for the identification of compounds with therapeutic potential in a broader range of conditions. Phenotypic screening expands the scope of drug repositioning opportunities but can sometimes fall short in terms of mechanism clarity. These methods not only discover repositioned drugs but also serve as a validation for drugs identified by computational models.

4.1 Binding assays

Binding assays are pivotal tools in drug repositioning, facilitating the identification of new therapeutic uses for existing drugs by evaluating their affinity for various biological targets. Proteomic techniques such as affinity chromatography and mass spectrometry are employed to identify the binding partners of drugs, facilitating the exploration of drug mechanisms and repositioning opportunities. The Cellular Thermostability Assay (CETSA) is another method that maps drug-target interactions within cells by detecting the thermal stabilization of proteins induced by drug-like ligands with suitable cellular affinity [54]. These assays provide a foundation for target validation in chemical biology, enhancing our understanding of a drug's therapeutic potential and aiding in the development of repurposed therapies.

4.2 Phenotypic screening

In contrast to binding assays, which rely on a confirmed association between molecular target and disease, phenotypic screening emphasizes the direct assessment of compounds' effects on biological systems associated with the disease, without presupposing the involvement of particular molecular targets. The most suitable biological system for phenotypic screening would involve humans. However, for ethical and safety reasons, this method is no longer considered viable. Model systems offer an alternative for phenotypic screening, including *in vitro* and *in vivo* phenotypic screening.

Typically, cell-based models are the most commonly used model systems. It leverages disease-related cells to explore a broad spectrum of potential drug activities. For example, based on the characteristics of Alzheimer's disease, Fischer et al. [82] used multiple cell lines to screen a library of extracts from plants to identify drug candidates for Alzheimer's disease. One of these extracts was demonstrated to possess potent neuroprotective and anti-inflammatory properties.

Complementing the cell-based models, the advancement of organoid models, which simulate the functions of a basic organ, has significantly enhanced the phenotypic screening methodology. Organoids are derived from stem cells and can self-organize into complex tissue structures, providing a valuable tool for disease modeling and drug testing [83]. Organoids can be used for drug repositioning screening in a variety of diseases. The key to using organoids for drug phenotypic screening is to develop organoid models that closely mimic the original disease state. In one such study, Saito et al. [84] successfully established organoids from biliary tract carcinoma (BTC) patients and repositioned antifungal drugs as potential therapeutic agents. And more recently, Mao et al. [85] established human colorectal cancer-derived organoids that well represent both morphological and molecular heterogeneities of original tumors. With this model, 335 drugs were tested and 34 drugs with anti-colorectal cancer effects were identified.

In vivo models utilize small animal models for phenotypic screening. These *in vivo* systems allow for the examination of intricate signaling pathways and interactions between tissues that cell-based models cannot replicate, thereby providing a more comprehensive understanding of drug effects. Considering the cost-effectiveness, *in vivo* screening is often combined with *in vitro* screening. Through a multi-faceted screening approach that includes high-throughput *in vitro* and *in vivo* phenotypic assessments, Lee et al. [86] have discovered XL888, an HSP90 inhibitor, to be an effective agent against tissue fibrosis by exhibiting potent senolytic properties.

5. Progress and challenges for drug repositioning in the AI-driven era

Drug repositioning offers significant advantages in pharmaceutical development by leveraging existing drugs for novel therapeutic purposes. Several classic examples highlight the success of drug repositioning across various diseases. For instance, sildenafil citrate, originally investigated as an antihypertensive, found unprecedented success when repurposed for erectile dysfunction due to its vasodilatory effects. Similarly, thalidomide, infamous for its historical association with birth defects, was repurposed first for erythema nodosum leprosum and later for multiple myeloma, demonstrating unexpected therapeutic benefits beyond its original indication [1]. These successes often stem from retrospective analyses and clinical observations rather than systematic approaches [54]. Clinical experiences and pharmacological insights into a drug's mechanisms of action have frequently guided these repositioning efforts. More FDA-approved repurposed drugs can be found in **Table 4**.

Future advancements in drug repositioning may harness AI for more systematic approaches. AI algorithms can sift through vast datasets to identify novel therapeutic uses and potential drug combinations, promising to accelerate the discovery process. While AI presents unprecedented opportunities, it also introduces a unique set of challenges that must be navigated to harness its full potential. We discuss these challenges and future prospects in this section.

5.1 Data issues

AI's voracious appetite for data necessitates the aggregation of vast and diverse datasets. The quality, standardization, and interoperability of these datasets are paramount for the development of reliable AI models. However, the heterogeneity and noise inherent in biomedical data can impede the performance of AI algorithms. Furthermore, the ethical considerations surrounding data privacy and patient consent become more pronounced in the digital age, demanding robust frameworks to ensure data security and compliance with regulations.

5.2 Computational modeling

The complexity of biological systems and the high dimensionality of omics data require advanced AI techniques such as deep learning and machine learning. These methods, while powerful, can be computationally intensive and may require significant expertise to implement effectively. While certain models may perform well on specific datasets, their ability to generalize to new or different datasets can be limited. There is a need for developing robust and adaptable models. Additionally, the "black box" nature of some AI models poses a challenge for regulatory approval and clinical acceptance, as the interpretability of AI-driven predictions is crucial for translating findings into clinical practice.

Drug	Original indications	New indications	Repositioning methods
Zidovudine	Cancer	HIV/AIDS	Phenotypic screening
Minoxidil	Hypertension	Hair loss	Retrospective clinical analysis
Rituximab	Various cancers	Rheumatoid arthritis	Retrospective clinical analysis
Raloxifene	Osteoporosis	Breast cancer	Retrospective clinical analysis
Topiramate	Epilepsy	Obesity	Pharmacological analysis
Ketoconazole	Fungal infections	Cushing syndrome	Pharmacological analysis
Aspirin	Analgesia	Colorectal cancer	Retrospective clinical and pharmacological analysis
Galantamine	Polio and muscle atrophy	Alzheimer's disease	Pharmacological analysis
Amantadine	Influenza A infection	Parkinson's disease	Case observation of a patient

Table 4.
Selected successful drug repositioning examples.

5.3 Regulatory and ethical considerations

The regulatory requirements and approval processes for drug repositioning may not be as well-defined as those for new drug development, leading to uncertainty for researchers and pharmaceutical companies in advancing repurposed drugs. The regulatory landscape for AI-driven drug repositioning is still evolving. The uncertainty in regulatory guidelines can create challenges for researchers and companies seeking to bring repurposed drugs to market. Moreover, ethical concerns regarding the use of AI in healthcare, such as potential biases in AI algorithms and the implications of personalized medicine, need to be addressed to build public trust and ensure equitable access to therapies.

5.4 Future prospects

Despite these challenges, the future of drug repositioning in the AI-driven era is promising. The development of more efficient algorithms, enhanced computational power, and innovative data integration techniques will likely overcome current data-driven hurdles. As AI models become more interpretable and their predictions more reliable, they will gain wider acceptance in the clinical and regulatory spheres. Furthermore, the ongoing dialog between the AI community, regulatory agencies, and ethicists will be instrumental in shaping guidelines that foster innovation while safeguarding patient welfare.

In conclusion, the AI-driven era presents both challenges and prospects for drug repositioning. By addressing data quality and privacy issues, enhancing computational methodologies, and working closely with regulatory bodies, the field can leverage AI to unlock new therapeutic opportunities and bring benefits to patients more rapidly than ever before. The road ahead requires a concerted effort from all stakeholders to ensure that AI serves as a catalyst for progress in drug repositioning.

6. Conclusion

This chapter has provided a comprehensive overview of drug repositioning in the AI-driven era, highlighting the profound impact of AI on accelerating drug discovery and the potential to uncover new therapeutic applications for existing drugs. We have explored the extensive use of biomedical databases, the evolution of computational methods from structure-based to machine-learning approaches, and the successful cases of drug repositioning across various diseases. The integration of AI with drug development has indeed marked a paradigm shift, enhancing the efficiency of drug repositioning through advanced data analysis and pattern recognition.

Looking ahead, while the field faces challenges such as data heterogeneity, computational complexity, and regulatory uncertainties, the future of AI in drug repositioning is promising. The development of more sophisticated algorithms, increased computational capabilities, and improved data integration strategies are set to overcome current hurdles. With enhanced transparency and improved reliability in their predictions, AI models are likely to gain wider acceptance in clinical practice and regulatory approval. In summary, the application of AI to drug repositioning holds great promise, offering the potential to revolutionize the way of drug repositioning and accelerate the delivery of novel therapies to patients in need.

Acknowledgements

This work was supported by National Key Research and Development Program of China (No.2023YFC2604400, No.2022YFA1103400); National Natural Science Foundation of China (No. 62103436); Beijing Nova Program (No.20230484454).

Conflict of interest

The authors declare no conflict of interest.

Author details

Jing Wang[1], Siming Kong[2], Xiaochen Bo[3], Yunfang Wang[2], Song He[3]* and Hui Bai[2]*

1 State Key Laboratory of Medicinal Chemical Biology, College of Pharmacy, Nankai University, Tianjin, China

2 Clinical Translational Research Center, Beijing Tsinghua Changgung Hospital, Tsinghua University, Beijing, China

3 Department of Biotechnology, Institute of Health Service and Transfusion Medicine, Beijing, China

*Address all correspondence to: hes1224@163.com and huibai13@hotmail.com; bha04160@btch.edu.cn

References

[1] Ashburn TT, Thor KB. Drug repositioning: Identifying and developing new uses for existing drugs. Nature Reviews. Drug Discovery. 2004;**3**:673-683. DOI: 10.1038/nrd1468

[2] Schwab RS, England AC Jr, Poskanzer DC, Young RR. Amantadine in the treatment of Parkinson's disease. Journal of the American Medical Association. 1969;**208**:1168-1170

[3] Cooke RM, Brown AJ, Marshall FH, Mason JS. Structures of G protein-coupled receptors reveal new opportunities for drug discovery. Drug Discovery Today. 2015;**20**:1355-1364. DOI: 10.1016/j.drudis.2015.08.003

[4] Dakshanamurthy S, Issa NT, Assefnia S, Seshasayee A, Peters OJ, Madhavan S, et al. Predicting new indications for approved drugs using a proteochemometric method. Journal of Medicinal Chemistry. 2012;**55**:6832-6848. DOI: 10.1021/jm300576q

[5] Kitchen DB, Decornez H, Furr JR, Bajorath J. Docking and scoring in virtual screening for drug discovery: Methods and applications. Nature Reviews. Drug Discovery. 2004;**3**:935-949. DOI: 10.1038/nrd1549

[6] Kumar S, Ayyannan SR. Identification of new small molecule monoamine oxidase-B inhibitors through pharmacophore-based virtual screening, molecular docking and molecular dynamics simulation studies. Journal of Biomolecular Structure and Dynamics. 2023;**41**:6789-6810. DOI: 10.1080/07391102.2022.2112082

[7] Abchir O, Khedraoui M, Nour H, Yamari I, Errougui A, Samadi A, et al. Integrative approach for designing novel triazole derivatives as α-glucosidase inhibitors: QSAR, molecular docking, ADMET, and molecular dynamics investigations. Pharmaceuticals. 2024;**17**:261

[8] Sadeghi M, Miroliaei M, Ghanadian M. Drug repurposing for diabetes mellitus: In silico and *in vitro* investigation of DrugBank database for alpha-glucosidase inhibitors. International Journal of Biological Macromolecules. 2024;**270**:132164. DOI: 10.1016/j.ijbiomac.2024.132164

[9] Chick JM, Munger SC, Simecek P, Huttlin EL, Choi K, Gatti DM, et al. Defining the consequences of genetic variation on a proteome-wide scale. Nature. 2016;**534**:500-505. DOI: 10.1038/nature18270

[10] Wainberg M, Sinnott-Armstrong N, Mancuso N, Barbeira AN, Knowles DA, Golan D, et al. Opportunities and challenges for transcriptome-wide association studies. Nature Genetics. 2019;**51**:592-599. DOI: 10.1038/s41588-019-0385-z

[11] Wang L, Lu Y, Li D, Zhou Y, Yu L, Mesa Eguiagaray I, et al. The landscape of the methodology in drug repurposing using human genomic data: A systematic review. Briefings in Bioinformatics. 2024;**25**:bbad527. DOI: 10.1093/bib/bbad527

[12] Iorio F, Rittman T, Ge H, Menden M, Saez-Rodriguez J. Transcriptional data: A new gateway to drug repositioning? Drug Discovery Today. 2013;**18**:350-357. DOI: 10.1016/j.drudis.2012.07.014

[13] Iorio F, Bosotti R, Scacheri E, Belcastro V, Mithbaokar P, Ferriero R, et al. Discovery of drug mode of action and drug repositioning from

transcriptional responses. Proceedings of the National Academy of Sciences of the United States of America. 2010;**107**:14621-14626. DOI: 10.1073/pnas.1000138107

[14] Wang Y, Guo M, Ren Y, Jia L, Yu G. Drug repositioning based on individual bi-random walks on a heterogeneous network. BMC Bioinformatics. 2019;**20**:547. DOI: 10.1186/s12859-019-3117-6

[15] Kim Y, Jung YS, Park JH, Kim SJ, Cho YR. Drug-disease association prediction using heterogeneous networks for computational drug repositioning. Biomolecules. 2022;**12**:1497. DOI: 10.3390/biom12101497

[16] Zhou X, Dai E, Song Q, Ma X, Meng Q, Jiang Y, et al. In silico drug repositioning based on drug-miRNA associations. Briefings in Bioinformatics. 2020;**21**:498-510. DOI: 10.1093/bib/bbz012

[17] Senior AW, Evans R, Jumper J, Kirkpatrick J, Sifre L, Green T, et al. Improved protein structure prediction using potentials from deep learning. Nature. 2020;**577**:706-710. DOI: 10.1038/s41586-019-1923-7

[18] Abramson J, Adler J, Dunger J, Evans R, Green T, Pritzel A, et al. Accurate structure prediction of biomolecular interactions with AlphaFold 3. Nature. 2024;**630**:493-500. DOI: 10.1038/s41586-024-07487-w

[19] Jumper J, Evans R, Pritzel A, Green T, Figurnov M, Ronneberger O, et al. Highly accurate protein structure prediction with AlphaFold. Nature. 2021;**596**:583-589. DOI: 10.1038/s41586-021-03819-2

[20] Brown AS, Patel CJ. MeSHDD: Literature-based drug-drug similarity for drug repositioning. Journal of the American Medical Informatics Association. 2017;**24**:614-618. DOI: 10.1093/jamia/ocw142

[21] Chen H, King FJ, Zhou B, Wang Y, Canedy CJ, Hayashi J, et al. Drug target prediction through deep learning functional representation of gene signatures. Nature Communications. 2024;**15**:1853. DOI: 10.1038/s41467-024-46089-y

[22] Shao K, Zhang Y, Wen Y, Zhang Z, He S, Bo X. DTI-HETA: Prediction of drug-target interactions based on GCN and GAT on heterogeneous graph. Briefings in Bioinformatics. 2022;**23**:bbac109. DOI: 10.1093/bib/bbac109

[23] Lee I, Keum J, Nam H. DeepConv-DTI: Prediction of drug-target interactions via deep learning with convolution on protein sequences. PLoS Computational Biology. 2019;**15**:e1007129. DOI: 10.1371/journal.pcbi.1007129

[24] Cheng X, Dai C, Wen Y, Wang X, Bo X, He S, et al. NeRD: A multichannel neural network to predict cellular response of drugs by integrating multidimensional data. BMC Medicine. 2022;**20**:368. DOI: 10.1186/s12916-022-02549-0

[25] Kuenzi BM, Park J, Fong SH, Sanchez KS, Lee J, Kreisberg JF, et al. Predicting drug response and synergy using a deep learning model of human cancer cells. Cancer Cell. 2020;**38**:672-684.e676. DOI: 10.1016/j.ccell.2020.09.014

[26] Sada Del Real K, Rubio A. Discovering the mechanism of action of drugs with a sparse explainable network. eBioMedicine. 2023;**95**:104767. DOI: 10.1016/j.ebiom.2023.104767

[27] Wu L, Gao J, Zhang Y, Sui B, Wen Y, Wu Q, et al. A hybrid deep forest-based method for predicting synergistic drug combinations. Cell Reports Methods. 2023;**3**:100411. DOI: 10.1016/j.crmeth.2023.100411

[28] Wu L, Wen Y, Leng D, Zhang Q, Dai C, Wang Z, et al. Machine learning methods, databases and tools for drug combination prediction. Briefings in Bioinformatics. 2022;**23**:bbab355. DOI: 10.1093/bib/bbab355

[29] Sun W, Sanderson PE, Zheng W. Drug combination therapy increases successful drug repositioning. Drug Discovery Today. 2016;**21**:1189-1195. DOI: 10.1016/j.drudis.2016.05.015

[30] Law V, Knox C, Djoumbou Y, Jewison T, Guo AC, Liu Y, et al. DrugBank 4.0: Shedding new light on drug metabolism. Nucleic Acids Research. 2014;**42**:D1091-D1097. DOI: 10.1093/nar/gkt1068

[31] Kim S, Thiessen PA, Bolton EE, Chen J, Fu G, Gindulyte A, et al. PubChem substance and compound databases. Nucleic Acids Research. 2016;**44**:D1202-D1213. DOI: 10.1093/nar/gkv951

[32] Liu H, Zhang W, Zou B, Wang J, Deng Y, Deng L. DrugCombDB: A comprehensive database of drug combinations toward the discovery of combinatorial therapy. Nucleic Acids Research. 2020;**48**:D871-d881. DOI: 10.1093/nar/gkz1007

[33] Gaulton A, Bellis LJ, Bento AP, Chambers J, Davies M, Hersey A, et al. ChEMBL: A large-scale bioactivity database for drug discovery. Nucleic Acids Research. 2012;**40**:D1100-D1107. DOI: 10.1093/nar/gkr777

[34] Kuhn M, Letunic I, Jensen LJ, Bork P. The SIDER database of drugs and side effects. Nucleic Acids Research. 2016;**44**:D1075-D1079. DOI: 10.1093/nar/gkv1075

[35] Zheng S, Aldahdooh J, Shadbahr T, Wang Y, Aldahdooh D, Bao J, et al. DrugComb update: A more comprehensive drug sensitivity data repository and analysis portal. Nucleic Acids Research. 2021;**49**:W174-w184. DOI: 10.1093/nar/gkab438

[36] UniProt Consortium. UniProt: A hub for protein information. Nucleic Acids Research. 2015;**43**:D204-D212. DOI: 10.1093/nar/gku989

[37] Velankar S, Best C, Beuth B, Boutselakis CH, Cobley N, Sousa Da Silva AW, et al. PDBe: Protein data bank in Europe. Nucleic Acids Research. 2010;**38**:D308-D317. DOI: 10.1093/nar/gkp916

[38] Harris MA, Clark J, Ireland A, Lomax J, Ashburner M, Foulger R, et al. The gene ontology (GO) database and informatics resource. Nucleic Acids Research. 2004;**32**:D258-D261. DOI: 10.1093/nar/gkh036

[39] Kanehisa M, Furumichi M, Tanabe M, Sato Y, Morishima K. KEGG: New perspectives on genomes, pathways, diseases and drugs. Nucleic Acids Research. 2017;**45**:D353-D361. DOI: 10.1093/nar/gkw1092

[40] Stark C, Breitkreutz BJ, Reguly T, Boucher L, Breitkreutz A, Tyers M. BioGRID: A general repository for interaction datasets. Nucleic Acids Research. 2006;**34**:D535-D539. DOI: 10.1093/nar/gkj109

[41] Keshava Prasad TS, Goel R, Kandasamy K, Keerthikumar S, Kumar S, Mathivanan S, et al. Human protein reference database--2009 update. Nucleic Acids Research. 2009;**37**:D767-D772. DOI: 10.1093/nar/gkn892

[42] von Mering C, Huynen M, Jaeggi D, Schmidt S, Bork P, Snel B. STRING: A database of predicted functional associations between proteins. Nucleic Acids Research. 2003;**31**:258-261. DOI: 10.1093/nar/gkg034

[43] Pinero J, Bravo A, Queralt-Rosinach N, Gutierrez-Sacristan A, Deu-Pons J, Centeno E, et al. DisGeNET: A comprehensive platform integrating information on human disease-associated genes and variants. Nucleic Acids Research. 2017;**45**:D833-D839. DOI: 10.1093/nar/gkw943

[44] Schriml LM, Munro JB, Schor M, Olley D, McCracken C, Felix V, et al. The human disease ontology 2022 update. Nucleic Acids Research. 2022;**50**:D1255-D1261. DOI: 10.1093/nar/gkab1063

[45] Kohler S, Gargano M, Matentzoglu N, Carmody LC, Lewis-Smith D, Vasilevsky NA, et al. The human phenotype ontology in 2021. Nucleic Acids Research. 2021;**49**:D1207-D1217. DOI: 10.1093/nar/gkaa1043

[46] Subramanian A, Narayan R, Corsello SM, Peck DD, Natoli TE, Lu X, et al. A next generation connectivity map: L1000 platform and the first 1,000,000 profiles. Cell. 2017;**171**(1437-1452):e1417. DOI: 10.1016/j.cell.2017.10.049

[47] Yang W, Soares J, Greninger P, Edelman EJ, Lightfoot H, Forbes S, et al. Genomics of drug sensitivity in cancer (GDSC): A resource for therapeutic biomarker discovery in cancer cells. Nucleic Acids Research. 2013;**41**:D955-D961. DOI: 10.1093/nar/gks1111

[48] Fang J, Zhang P, Zhou Y, Chiang CW, Tan J, Hou Y, et al. Endophenotype-based in silico network medicine discovery combined with insurance record data mining identifies sildenafil as a candidate drug for Alzheimer's disease. Nature Aging. 2021;**1**:1175-1188. DOI: 10.1038/s43587-021-00138-z

[49] Lamb J, Crawford ED, Peck D, Modell JW, Blat IC, Wrobel MJ, et al. The connectivity map: Using gene-expression signatures to connect small molecules, genes, and disease. Science. 2006;**313**:1929-1935. DOI: 10.1126/science.1132939

[50] Tang B, Wang Y, Jiang X, Thambisetty M, Ferrucci L, Johnell K, et al. Genetic variation in targets of antidiabetic drugs and Alzheimer disease risk: A Mendelian randomization study. Neurology. 2022;**99**:e650-e659. DOI: 10.1212/wnl.0000000000200771

[51] Wang X, He S, Zhou Z, Bo X, Qi D, Fu X, et al. LINCS dataset-based repositioning of rosiglitazone as a potential anti-human adenovirus drug. Antiviral Research. 2020;**179**:104789. DOI: 10.1016/j.antiviral.2020.104789

[52] Liu X, Wang S, Meng F, Wang J, Zhang Y, Dai E, et al. SM2miR: A database of the experimentally validated small molecules' effects on microRNA expression. Bioinformatics. 2013;**29**:409-411. DOI: 10.1093/bioinformatics/bts698

[53] Barretina J, Caponigro G, Stransky N, Venkatesan K, Margolin AA, Kim S, et al. The cancer cell line encyclopedia enables predictive modelling of anticancer drug sensitivity. Nature. 2012;**483**:603-607. DOI: 10.1038/nature11003

[54] Pushpakom S, Iorio F, Eyers PA, Escott KJ, Hopper S, Wells A, et al. Drug repurposing: Progress, challenges and recommendations. Nature Reviews. Drug Discovery. 2019;**18**:41-58. DOI: 10.1038/nrd.2018.168

[55] Morris GM, Huey R, Lindstrom W, Sanner MF, Belew RK, Goodsell DS, et al. AutoDock4 and AutoDockTools4: Automated docking with selective receptor flexibility. Journal of Computational Chemistry. 2009;**30**:2785-2791. DOI: 10.1002/jcc.21256

[56] Jones G, Willett P, Glen RC, Leach AR, Taylor R. Development and validation of a genetic algorithm for flexible docking. Journal of Molecular Biology. 1997;**267**:727-748. DOI: 10.1006/jmbi.1996.0897

[57] Kramer B, Rarey M, Lengauer T. Evaluation of the FLEXX incremental construction algorithm for protein-ligand docking. Proteins. 1999;**37**:228-241. DOI: 10.1002/(sici)1097-0134(19991101)37:2<228::aid-prot8>3.0.co;2-8

[58] Jain AN. Surflex: Fully automatic flexible molecular docking using a molecular similarity-based search engine. Journal of Medicinal Chemistry. 2003;**46**:499-511. DOI: 10.1021/jm020406h

[59] Friesner RA, Banks JL, Murphy RB, Halgren TA, Klicic JJ, Mainz DT, et al. Glide: A new approach for rapid, accurate docking and scoring. 1. Method and assessment of docking accuracy. Journal of Medicinal Chemistry. 2004;**47**:1739-1749. DOI: 10.1021/jm0306430

[60] Kharkar PS, Warrier S, Gaud RS. Reverse docking: A powerful tool for drug repositioning and drug rescue. Future Medicinal Chemistry. 2014;**6**:333-342. DOI: 10.4155/fmc.13.207

[61] Pagadala NS, Syed K, Tuszynski J. Software for molecular docking: A review. Biophysical Reviews. 2017;**9**:91-102. DOI: 10.1007/s12551-016-0247-1

[62] Warren GL, Andrews CW, Capelli AM, Clarke B, LaLonde J, Lambert MH, et al. A critical assessment of docking programs and scoring functions. Journal of Medicinal Chemistry. 2006;**49**:5912-5931. DOI: 10.1021/jm050362n

[63] Alonso H, Bliznyuk AA, Gready JE. Combining docking and molecular dynamic simulations in drug design. Medicinal Research Reviews. 2006;**26**:531-568. DOI: 10.1002/med.20067

[64] Dehghan A. Genome-wide association studies. Methods in Molecular Biology. 2018;**1793**:37-49. DOI: 10.1007/978-1-4939-7868-7_4

[65] Chen F, Wang X, Jang SK, Quach BC, Weissenkampen JD, Khunsriraksakul C, et al. Multi-ancestry transcriptome-wide association analyses yield insights into tobacco use biology and drug repurposing. Nature Genetics. 2023;**55**:291-300. DOI: 10.1038/s41588-022-01282-x

[66] Imami AS, McCullumsmith RE, O'Donovan SM. Strategies to identify candidate repurposable drugs: COVID-19 treatment as a case example. Translational Psychiatry. 2021;**11**:591. DOI: 10.1038/s41398-021-01724-w

[67] Koudijs KKM, van Scheltinga AGTT, Böhringer S, Schimmel KJM, Guchelaar HJ. Transcriptome signature reversion as a method to reposition drugs against cancer for precision oncology. Cancer Journal. 2019;**25**:116-120. DOI: 10.1097/Ppo.0000000000000370

[68] Iorio F, Isacchi A, di Bernardo D, Brunetti-Pierri N. Identification of small molecules enhancing autophagic function from drug network analysis. Autophagy. 2010;**6**:1204-1205. DOI: 10.1073/pnas.1000138107

[69] Jarada TN, Rokne JG, Alhajj R. A review of computational drug

repositioning: Strategies, approaches, opportunities, challenges, and directions. Journal of Cheminformatics. 2020;**12**:46. DOI: 10.1186/s13321-020-00450-7

[70] Li T, Zhao XM, Li L. Co-VAE: Drug-target binding affinity prediction by co-regularized variational autoencoders. IEEE Transactions on Pattern Analysis and Machine Intelligence. 2022;**44**:8861-8873. DOI: 10.1109/TPAMI.2021.3120428

[71] Pan F, Yin C, Liu SQ, Huang T, Bian Z, Yuen PC. BindingSiteDTI: Differential-scale binding site modelling for drug-target interaction prediction. Bioinformatics. 2024;**40**:btae308. DOI: 10.1093/bioinformatics/btae308

[72] Liu H, Zhang W, Song Y, Deng L, Zhou S. HNet-DNN: Inferring new drug-disease associations with deep neural network based on heterogeneous network features. Journal of Chemical Information and Modeling. 2020;**60**:2367-2376. DOI: 10.1021/acs.jcim.9b01008

[73] Meng Y, Wang Y, Xu J, Lu C, Tang X, Peng T, et al. Drug repositioning based on weighted local information augmented graph neural network. Briefings in Bioinformatics. 2023;**25**:bbad431. DOI: 10.1093/bib/bbad431

[74] Ma J, Fong SH, Luo Y, Bakkenist CJ, Shen JP, Mourragui S, et al. Few-shot learning creates predictive models of drug response that translate from high-throughput screens to individual patients. Nature Cancer. 2021;**2**:233-244. DOI: 10.1038/s43018-020-00169-2

[75] Wang H, Dai C, Wen Y, Wang X, Liu W, He S, et al. GADRP: Graph convolutional networks and autoencoders for cancer drug response prediction. Briefings in Bioinformatics. 2023;**24**:bbac501. DOI: 10.1093/bib/bbac501

[76] So E, Yu F, Wang B, Haibe-Kains B. Reusability report: Evaluating reproducibility and reusability of a fine-tuned model to predict drug response in cancer patient samples. Nature Machine Intelligence. 2023;**5**:792-798. DOI: 10.1038/s42256-023-00688-4

[77] Xie L, He S, Zhang Z, Lin K, Bo X, Yang S, et al. Domain-adversarial multi-task framework for novel therapeutic property prediction of compounds. Bioinformatics. 2020;**36**:2848-2855. DOI: 10.1093/bioinformatics/btaa063

[78] Dong J, Wang NN, Yao ZJ, Zhang L, Cheng Y, Ouyang D, et al. ADMETlab: A platform for systematic ADMET evaluation based on a comprehensively collected ADMET database. Journal of Cheminformatics. 2018;**10**:29. DOI: 10.1186/s13321-018-0283-x

[79] Xiong G, Wu Z, Yi J, Fu L, Yang Z, Hsieh C, et al. ADMETlab 2.0: An integrated online platform for accurate and comprehensive predictions of ADMET properties. Nucleic Acids Research. 2021;**49**:W5-w14. DOI: 10.1093/nar/gkab255

[80] Fu L, Shi S, Yi J, Wang N, He Y, Wu Z, et al. ADMETlab 3.0: An updated comprehensive online ADMET prediction platform enhanced with broader coverage, improved performance, API functionality and decision support. Nucleic Acids Research. 2024;**52**(W1):W422-W431. DOI: 10.1093/nar/gkae236

[81] Janizek JD, Dincer AB, Celik S, Chen H, Chen W, Naxerova K, et al. Uncovering expression signatures of synergistic drug responses via ensembles of explainable machine-learning models. Nature Biomedical Engineering.

2023;**7**:811-829. DOI: 10.1038/s41551-023-01034-0

[82] Fischer W, Currais A, Liang Z, Pinto A, Maher P. Old age-associated phenotypic screening for Alzheimer's disease drug candidates identifies sterubin as a potent neuroprotective compound from yerba santa. Redox Biology. 2019;**21**:101089. DOI: 10.1016/j.redox.2018.101089

[83] Han X, Cai C, Deng W, Shi Y, Li L, Wang C, et al. Landscape of human organoids: Ideal model in clinics and research. Innovation (Camb). 2024;**5**:100620. DOI: 10.1016/j.xinn.2024.100620

[84] Saito Y, Muramatsu T, Kanai Y, Ojima H, Sukeda A, Hiraoka N, et al. Establishment of patient-derived organoids and drug screening for biliary tract carcinoma. Cell Reports. 2019;**27**:1265-1276.e1264. DOI: 10.1016/j.celrep.2019.03.088

[85] Mao Y, Wang W, Yang J, Zhou X, Lu Y, Gao J, et al. Drug repurposing screening and mechanism analysis based on human colorectal cancer organoids. Protein & Cell. 2024;**15**:285-304. DOI: 10.1093/procel/pwad038

[86] Lee JY, Reyes NS, Ravishankar S, Zhou M, Krasilnikov M, Ringler C, et al. An in vivo screening platform identifies senolytic compounds that target p16INK4a+ fibroblasts in lung fibrosis. The Journal of Clinical Investigation. 2024;**134**:e173371. DOI: 10.1172/jci173371

Section 2

Specific Topics

Chapter 4

Advantages, Challenges, and Impact of Drug Repurposing for Cancer Treatment

Rabia Zafar, Iqra Safdar, Aaiza Munir, Maah Rukh Zahid and Saad Serfraz

Abstract

Drug repurposing involves identifying new therapeutic uses for existing drugs, offering a cost-effective and time-efficient alternative to traditional drug discovery against cancer. Key approaches include computational, experimental, and drug-centric strategies, which have demonstrated success in targeting specific cancer types such as colorectal cancer with aspirin and BCC with itraconazole. Additionally, repurposing has shown potential in combination therapies, enhancing treatment efficacy, preventing metastasis, disrupting metabolic processes in cancer cells, improving cancer immunotherapy, and overcoming resistance mechanisms. Despite its benefits, drug repurposing faces significant obstacles, including cancer's biological complexity, clinical trial design challenges, intellectual property barriers, biases affecting repurposing outcomes, and access to knowledge. Cancer heterogeneity complicates the development of universally effective therapies, while high costs and regulatory hurdles of clinical trials hinder rapid advancement. Furthermore, limited patent incentives reduce industry interest in repurposing projects. AI is revolutionizing drug repurposing by identifying new therapeutic targets and predicting drug interactions, yet challenges related to data quality, interpretability, and computational requirements necessitate careful integration. To overcome these barriers, collaboration between academia, industry, and regulatory bodies, alongside innovations in bioinformatics and clinical trial methodologies, is critical for advancing drug repurposing as a viable strategy for cancer treatment. This chapter explore the advantages, impacts, and challenges of drug repurposing in oncology, emphasizing its potential to accelerate the development of effective therapies while navigating obstacles such as data quality, regulatory challenges, and the necessity for comprehensive clinical validation.

Keywords: cancer, drug repurposing, combination therapy, drug resistance, computational drug discovery, cancer metastasis prevention, bioinformatics tools, artificial intelligence

1. Introduction

Drug repurposing or reprofiling is a strategy to identifying new therapeutic uses for existing drugs with suitable safety and pharmacokinetic properties [1]. Drug repurposing, a multi-faceted drug discovery landscape, has been sought to explore novel indications thereby addressing high unmet medical needs, particularly in diseases that are chronic and economically infeasible to develop new drugs [2]. Traditional drug discovery is an expensive and time-consuming process. This process typically involves the discovery and preclinical testing of the compound, its safety evaluation, clinical research, approval from FDA and post market monitoring. However, drug repurposing involves assessing approved drug library, drug target analysis, clinical trials and post market safety monitoring [3]. Furthermore, the introduction of computational biology, artificial intelligence (AI), and bioinformatics is contributing to more accurate identification of novel drug indications for existing drugs which in turn systematically accelerates the repurposing process [4]. Rapid advancements in bioinformatics have significantly reduced the time required for drug repurposing, allowing researchers to identify the new drug targets within 1 to 2 years and complete the full development of a repurposed drug in approximately 8 years [3] (**Figure 1**).

Cancer remains a major health concern and is one of the leading causes of death globally [5]. In 2020, global cancer statistics estimate 19.3 million new cases of cancer and approximately 10.0 million cancer-related deaths [6]. Clinicians face significant challenges in treating various types of cancer [7]. Developing new cancer medicine is a long and complex process with the approval process often taking several years or even decades. For example, Gleevec the first therapeutic kinase inhibitor, took over a decade to become the standard treatment for chronic myeloid leukemia (CML), a condition affecting roughly 0.2% of the population during their lifetime. The timeline for drug approval can be even longer for treatments targeting smaller patient populations or those with less definitive therapeutic outcomes. Another example is omacetaxine, that inhibit protein translation, took more than 30 years to be approved to treat tyrosine kinase inhibitors (TKI)-resistant CML [8]. However, drug repurposing has emerged as an alternative strategy for developing antitumor drugs. Consequently, repurposed drugs can expedite the transition from preclinical and Phase I clinical trials to Phase II and III studies, with an increased likelihood of successful progression through the clinical trial stages. This approach can potentially shorten the research

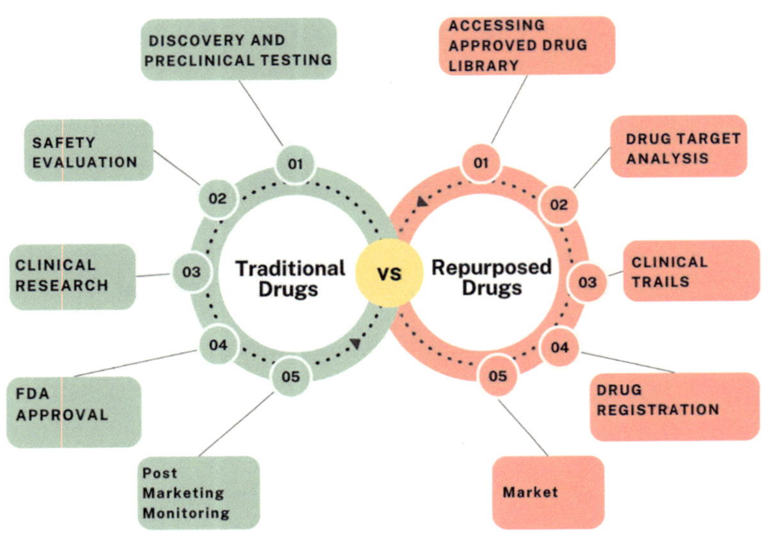

Figure 1.
Traditional vs. repurposed drug.

and development cycle by 3 to 5 years and reduce associated costs by approximately 0.3 billion dollar [9]. It has been proposed that up to 75% of existing medications can be repositioned for various chronic or rare diseases [10].

2. Drug repurposing approaches for cancer treatment

Drug repurposing employs three different types of approaches: mixed approaches, experimental approaches, and computational approaches. Experimental repurposing strategies use dynamic approaches like phenotypic screening and binding assays, to identify new leads [11, 12]. However, by using computational techniques, scientific evidence from multiple biological datasets can be integrated to infer new drug-disease interactions through bioinformatics, and network or systems biology approaches. These approaches take advantage of extensive chemical libraries and high-throughput screening (HTS) to identify novel repurposing candidates more efficiently [13].

2.1 Experimental approaches

2.1.1 Binding assays

Binding assays measure how a drug interacts with its target, providing insights into new targets and therapeutic mechanisms. They are valuable for understanding the specificity and affinity of drug-target interactions, which can reveal new indications for existing drugs [11]. Proteomic approaches, such as mass spectrometry and affinity chromatography, have helped to identify drug binding partners and characterizing these interactions [14]. A notable technique, cellular thermal shift assay (CETSA), utilizes the principles of thermal stabilization to map drug interactions with target proteins within living cells. CETSA has been successfully employed to validate the binding of drugs like crizotinib and acetaminophen to their respective cellular targets [15]. Therefore, experimentations proposed that chemical genetics can help connect binding to function in cells [16]. The findings can rapidly translate into new clinical applications and are particularly valuable in overcoming resistance mechanisms of kinase inhibitor therapy in cancer. For instance, kinase inhibitors such as sorafenib and dasatinib have shown unexpected potency against non-primary kinase targets, for example, BRAF/REKIN [17].

2.1.2 Phenotypic drug-screening

Phenotypic screening involves searches through very large libraries to identify lead compounds with effective biological activities, often leading to unexpected discovery [12]. It is a valuable strategy of finding drugs without requiring prior knowledge about molecular targets that cause disease-relevant effects in model systems. This approach is particularly effective in highlighting drug repurposing opportunities, especially for compounds already known or under development for other therapeutic indications. For example, a library of small molecules was tested in multiple prostate cancer cell and normal cell lines. This screening identified disulfiram (DSF), traditionally used to treat alcoholism, as a promising anti-cancer agent. The potential of DSF in cancer treatment was subsequently confirmed through gene expression analyses, underscoring its repurposing potential in oncology [18].

2.2 Computational approaches

2.2.1 Signature matching

Signature matching is a computational technique for the identification of novel therapeutic uses of existing drugs or to uncover off-target effects. This approach utilizes transcriptomic, metabolomic, and proteomic data to compare biological profiles across various states, including healthy, disease-associated, and medication-treated conditions [19]. By comparative transcriptomics, signature matching can provide insights into drug-drug and drug-disease interactions [20, 21]. Transcriptomic matching relies heavily on the comparison of gene expression profiles, which are often sourced from publicly accessible databases [22]. By employing advanced computational techniques, we can analyze disease signatures alongside connectivity map data for identification of new associations between drug and disease and explore potential drug repurposing opportunities [23]. Metabolomics focuses on analyzing metabolic changes, providing insights into possible therapeutic targets and offering a detailed molecular perspective of disease and treatment [24]. Proteomics, on the other hand, studies drug-protein interactions, offering valuable information on drug safety, toxicity, and mechanisms of action. Together, these approaches provide a comprehensive view of a drug's effects across genetic, metabolic, and proteomic spectra, enhancing our understanding of therapeutic interventions and their potential for repurposing [25].

2.2.2 Drug-centric approaches

Drug-centric strategies focus on repurposing existing drugs by studying their pleiotropic mechanism of targets. These strategies often involve polypharmacological drugs which, despite their potential for side effects, opens the door to exploring new therapeutic indications through multiple targets [26]. The discovery involves the evaluation of drug-receptor interactions, particularly for off-target effects. By investigating drug-target binding as well as structurally related molecules, novel medicinal applications can be uncovered from repositories. One notable tool in this domain is RepurposeVS, which is renowned for its ability to predict drug-protein interactions. This tool has been particularly effective in identifying anti-neoplastic agents with significant repurposing potential [27].

2.2.3 Target-based approaches

Target repositioning involves repurposing a drug to act on the same molecular target but for a different disease and off-target repositioning involves utilizing an existing drug against a different type of disease through its secondary mechanisms of action [28]. This strategy is very popular, and about 80% of all drug repurposing projects rely on this [29].

3. Major advantages of drug repurposing in cancer treatment

3.1 Drug repurposing led to faster development and cost effectiveness

Drug repurposing offers significant advantages in cancer treatment, particularly when compared to traditional drug discovery processes. The development of new drug is often a costly and time-consuming process, typically requiring 10–17 years and costing millions of dollars. Additionally, the process is characterized by a high attrition rate, with approximately 90% of drug candidate being discarded due to safety and efficacy concerns [30]. However, repurposed drugs are generally cost-effective and can reduce the time required for drug development process due to their prior approval, known safety, and reduced risk of failure [31]. A notable example of drug repurposing is thalidomide, initially developed as a sedative, withdrawn from the market due to its tragic teratogenic effects, which led to skeletal deformities in infants born to mothers who took the drug during their first trimester [11, 32]. However, in 1964, thalidomide was found to be effective in treating a severe complication of leprosy called erythema nodosum leprosum (ENL) [33]. This unexpected discovery marked a significant shift in the drug's use. Subsequently, thalidomide has also been shown to be highly effective in the treatment of cancer, particularly multiple myeloma [34]. Thalidomide and its derivative lenalidomide have become standard treatments for multiple myeloma significantly to improve the outcomes and survival rates of patients. The repurposing of thalidomide was notably faster and more cost effective than developing a new drug as its safety and pharmacological profile were already understood [35].

3.2 Drug repurposing for specific cancer types

The success of drug repurposing in specific cancer types highlights its potential to provide effective, accessible, and cost-efficient treatment options. For example, aspirin, a widely used anti-inflammatory drug primarily known for its role in preventing thrombotic cardiovascular diseases, has emerged as a promising chemopreventive agent in colorectal cancer. This suggests that regular aspirin use may reduce the colorectal cancer, which has led to ongoing clinical trials aimed at assessing its efficacy as a preventive measure in high-risk populations [36]. Another notable example is itraconazole, an antifungal drug found to inhibit hedgehog signaling pathway, which is critical in the development of basal cell carcinoma (BCC). In a clinical trial, treatment with itraconazole result a significant reduction in both tumor cell growth and Hedgehog pathway activity, with an average 24% reduction in tumor size. Furthermore, in patients with multiple tumors, some experienced partial tumor shrinkage, suggesting that itraconazole may be a valuable treatment option for BCC [37]. Similarly, propranolol which is originally developed as a beta-blocker for cardiovascular conditions has been repurposed for the treatment of angiosarcoma, showing significant tumor regression in clinical studies [38].

3.3 Drug repurposing for broader cancer treatment

Drug repurposing has demonstrated notable success in targeting specific cancer types and holds considerable promise for broader oncological applications. Metformin, a drug originally developed for the management of diabetes, has been identified as a potential inhibitor of cancer cell proliferation across various malignancies. Recent work indicates that metformin may enhance the efficacy of cancer therapies, particularly in breast and prostate cancers [39]. Specifically, metformin has been shown to reduce HER2 expression in human breast cancer (BC) cells [40]. In a murine model of tobacco carcinogen-induced lung cancer, metformin's inhibition of the insulin-like growth factor 1 receptor/insulin receptor led to diminished downstream signaling through the Akt pathway. This effect resulted in reduced mTOR activation

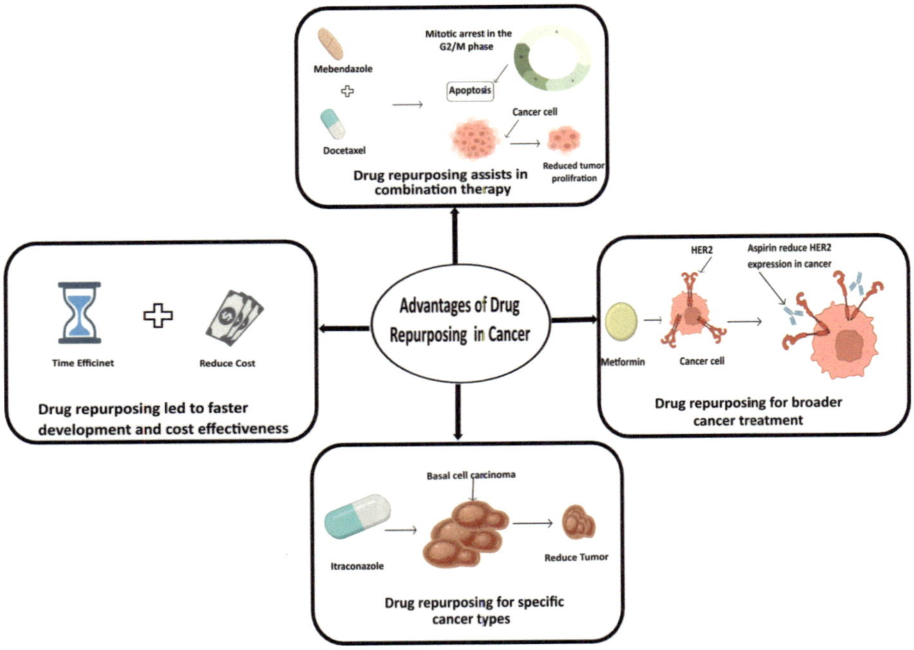

Figure 2.
Schematic representation of advantages of repurposing drugs in cancer. (3.1) Drug repurposing led to faster development and cost effectiveness. (3.2) Drug repurposing for specific cancer types (such as itraconazole for BCC, has shown efficacy in reducing tumor size and inhibiting Hedgehog pathway activity). (3.3) Drug repurposing for broader cancer treatment (e.g., metformin, which downregulates HER2 expression in BC cells). (3.4) Drug repurposing assists in combination therapy (e.g., MBZ in combination with docetaxel leading to tumor reduction and induction of apoptosis in prostate cancer).

within lung tissue and was associated with a 72% reduction in tumor burden [41]. Furthermore, metformin's impact on the AMPK signaling pathway plays an important role in inhibiting growth of cancer cells and metabolism, highlighting its potential as a valuable agent in the treatment of cancer (**Figure 2**) [42].

3.4 Drug repurposing assists in combination therapy

Targeted therapies in cancer treatment often exhibited reduced antitumor efficacy due to inherent and resistance mechanisms, emphasizing the need of rational combination therapies to achieve more effective responses [43]. Drug repurposing has emerged as a crucial strategy in the development of combination therapies to improve treatment efficacy and overcome resistance in cancer. For example, MBZ, a synthetic benzimidazole anthelmintic with established pharmacokinetic properties and a well-documented toxicity profile [44] when used in combination with temozolomide (TMZ), a standard treatment for malignant gliomas, significantly enhanced tumor suppression in both syngeneic and xenograft glioma models compared to TMZ monotherapy [45]. Additionally, MBZ and docetaxel showed synergistic effects by preventing tubulin polymerization, inducing mitotic arrest in G2/M phase, promoting apoptosis, and lowering prostate cancer cell proliferation, ultimately leading to tumor growth suppression [46]. Another example is the combination therapy of doxorubicin and selinexor which has been shown to synergistically induce cell death in both thyroid cancer cell and acute myeloid leukemia (AML) cells [47]. Similarly, the combined use of imatinib and clotrimazole has been found to more effectively inhibit the glycolysis pathway and enhance the production of vascular endothelial growth factor (VEGE) and nitric oxide in BC [48].

4. Impact of drug repurposing on cancer treatment

4.1 Enhancing therapeutic efficacy and safety

Drug repurposing offers multiple advantages, including reduced toxicity, enhanced therapeutic efficacy, the potential for dose reduction without compromising effectiveness, and overcoming resistance mechanisms commonly observed in existing cancer treatments [49]. Drug repurposing is a more economical and time-efficient approach than de novo drug development, significantly broadening the spectrum of clinically available cancer therapies [50]. Drug repurposing has shown significant value in the treatment of BC, a leading cause of mortality among women, due to its high metastatic potential and therapy resistance. The complexity and heterogeneity of BC, especially its subtypes such as triple negative BC, make the development of novel therapeutic agents a prolonged and costly process. However, in recent years, drugs originally developed for other conditions such as alcoholism, parasitic infections, and epilepsy have been repurposed to enhance the effectiveness of BC therapies. By targeting diverse molecular pathways, these repurposed drugs offer a more comprehensive and potentially more effective therapeutic strategy to combating this challenging disease [51].

4.2 Preventing tumor invasion and metastasis

Tumor invasion and metastasis are major contributors to cancer progression, leading to significant mortality. The epithelial-mesenchymal transition (EMT) is a key process in metastasis in cancer cells, and its aberrant activation is regulated by intricate signaling pathways [52]. Research has revealed that repurposing of drugs can effectively target these key signaling pathways, demonstrating potential antitumor activity across various metastatic cancer models [31]. For example, mebendazole (MBZ), originally an antiparasitic agent, has shown promising anticancer properties. It disrupts growth of tumor cells in several cancer cell lines by inhibiting microtubule polymerization. In addition to its antiproliferative effects, MBZ has been shown to suppress cancer cell invasion and metastasis [53] Specifically, MBZ decreases the invasive and migratory capabilities of glioblastoma cells, indicating its potential to limit the spread of highly aggressive cancers [54].

4.3 Metabolic regulation in cancer cells

The rapid proliferation of tumor cells is driven by metabolic changes which enables tumors to meet their increase energy demands [55]. Recent research has identified dysregulation of cellular energetics as a hallmark of cancer. Although, development of metabolism-targeted therapies of cancer has faced challenges, repurposing of drug offers a promising alternative approach. Preclinical studies have extensively explored repurposed drugs for their ability to target critical pathways in cancer metabolism, with some progressing to or nearing clinical trials. This highlights the potential impact of repurposing drug as an effective strategy to disrupt the metabolic processes that sustain cancer cell proliferation. Such as DSF, initially approved to treat alcoholism, has recently gained attention for its potent anticancer properties. Notably, DSF has been shown to alter cellular energy metabolism, making it a promising candidate in the context of cancer therapy [31].

4.4 Inhibiting tumor-associated inflammation

Tumor-associated inflammation is a critical factor in cancer progression, facilitating tumor growth, invasion and metastasis. This inflammation is driven by

Drug name	Original use	Repurposed	References
Auranofin	Rheumatoid arthritis	Ovarian cancer	[60]
Nelfinavir	HIV	Cervical cancer	[61]
Lovastatin	Hypercholesterolaemia	Breast cancer	[62]
Metformin	Diabetes	Prostrate and breast cancer	[39]
Mebendazole	Helminthic infections	Lung cancer	[45]
Aspirin	Pain and fever	Colon cancer	[46]
Telmisartan	Cardiovascular drug	Lung and gastric cancer	[63]
Capecitabine	Colon cancer	Breast cancer	[64]
Thalidomide	Sedative	Multiple myeloma	[35]
Azithromycin	Antibacterial	Colon and pulmonary cancer	[65, 66]
Rapamycin	Antifungal	Breast cancer	[67]
Quinacrine	Antimalarial	Renal cancer	[68]
Atovaquone	Antimalarial	Prostate, colon, and breast cancer	[69]
Losartan	Cardiovascular drugs	Glioblastoma and ovarian cancer	[70]
Benazepril	Cardiovascular drugs	Esophageal carcinoma	[71]
Ibuprofen	Anti-inflammatory drugs	Adenocarcinoma and lung cancer	[72]
Anastrazole	Ovulation induction	Breast cancer	[64]
Capecitabine	Colon cancer	Breast cancer	[64]
Flubendazol	Antihelmintic	Multiple myeloma	[73]
Eprinomectin	Antiprotozoal	Prostate cancer	[74]
Ribavirin	Antiviral	Squamous cell carcinoma	[75]
Cidofovir	Antiviral	Glioblastoma	[76]
Doxycycline	Antibiotics	Colon cancer	[77]
Griseofulvin	Antifungal	Colorectal cancer	[78]
Niclosamide	Antihelmintic	Prostate cancer	[79]
Ritonavir	HIV	Kaposis sarcoma	[80]
Berberine	Bacterial diarrhea	Colorectal cancer	[81]

The table shows how antimalarials, antibiotics, antifungals, and cardiovascular medicines have been effectively repurposed for many forms of cancer. Drug repurposing is becoming an increasingly essential method in modern drug discovery for cancer due to its ability to hasten the development of novel medicine while also expanding the therapeutic uses of current pharmaceutical.

Table 1.
List of some drugs that have been repurposed for new therapeutic indications beyond their original intended use.

the tumor microenvironment (TME), which recruits immune cells that instead of fighting the cancer, contribute to its development. Targeting these inflammatory pathways through drug repurposing has shown significant potential in inhibiting tumor growth. For example, celecoxib, a drug traditionally used to treat arthritis [56] has demonstrated significant potential in reducing tumor-associated inflammation, thereby inhibiting the growth of various tumors. The promising results from preclinical studies have led to an increase in clinical trials exploring the use of celecoxib in oncology, particularly in combination with immunotherapy and chemotherapy, to potentially enhance treatment outcomes. These findings underscore the strategic value of targeting inflammation in cancer therapy and highlight the potential of drug repurposing [31].

4.5 Enhancing cancer immunotherapy

In early tumorigenesis, lymphocytes like cytotoxic natural killer (NK) cells and T cells target tumor cells by inducing apoptosis through perforin and granzyme or the death ligand/receptor pathway [31]. However, as tumors progress, the TME becomes more immunosuppressive, with tumor cells expressing program death ligand 1 (PD-L1) to inhibit NK and T cell activity [57]. This, along with suppressive immune cell populations, diminishes natural antitumor immunity. Immunotherapies like immune checkpoint inhibitors and adoptive cell transfer aim to boost immune responses but are not universally effective. Consequently, there is increasing interest in repurposing drugs to activate antitumor immunity and enhance cancer treatment [31]. For instance, oleanolic acid (OA), known for its antiparasitic properties, has recently been studied for its impacts on antitumor immunity, suggesting that it may be a viable option for cancer treatment through drug repurposing (**Table 1**) [58, 59].

5. Challenges and future directions

Advancement of drug repurposing approach has been challenging due to cancer's biological complexity, clinical trial designing, lack of funding, and pharmaceutical industry interest [82]. Several major aspects contribute to cancer's complexity.

5.1 Biological complexity of cancer

Cancer is a complex disease spread via arteries, lymph nodes, and nerves, involving the entire body. Its defective genetic and epigenetic networks contribute to tumor formation [83]. Cancer is a diverse disease, exhibiting both genetic and phenotypic indications within individual tumors and between tumor of different types [84].

Heterogeneity, or variety in cancer cell morphology, transcriptional patterns, metabolism, and metastatic potential, is a universal issue in most tumors and a key barrier in cancer ecosystem [85]. This diversity induces varied reactions to medicines, accomplishing it difficult to develop repurposed medications that can strongly target all tumor subpopulations [86]. We can overthrow heterogeneity in drug repurposing by stratifying analysis, integrating multi-omics data, standardizing protocols, and ensuring via validation over diverse models and cohorts, identifying patient subgroups based on biomarkers and genetic factors [11].

The TME is a complicated system, includes stromal cells, endothelial cells, tumor cells, immune cells, and extracellular matrix components. Tumor cell invasion and metastasis require association with TME components, which affect critical incident such as tumor recurrence, metastasis, and immunotherapy reaction, all of which have an impact on clinical consequence [87]. The cooperation of cancer cells and the TME can cause adaptive resistance, in which tumors develop in response to therapy, lowering the effectiveness of repurposed drugs. To combat this concern, repurposed drugs can enhance conventional treatments by combining with anti-inflammatory drugs or immune modulators and targeting TME components like cancer-associated fibroblast (CAFs) or immune checkpoints can improve drug repurposing consequences [88].

Drug repurposing confers significant pharmacokinetic and pharmacodynamic challenges, as repurposed drugs may have reformed absorption, distribution, metabolism, and excretion (ADME) profile, and requires dose adjustments and drug delivery approach. One significant concern is the bioavailability and tissue distribution of repurposed medications, which may not acquire enough concentrations at the tumor site, limiting their therapeutic effectiveness [89]. To overcome pharmacokinetic and pharmacodynamic threat in drug repurposing, it is imperative to acclimate the drug's ADME profiles, adjusting dosing regimens and using advanced delivery methods to attain effective drug concentrations [90].

5.2 Clinical trial design: Challenges in designing appropriate trials for repurposed drugs

Repurposing projects often eliminate preclinical testing, but clinical trials are still necessary to illustrate effectiveness and protection in the target indication. Diversity of cancer patient populations, including multifactorial nature, genetic mutations, and prior treatments, makes standardizing trial design challenging. Trials' extent depends on available data and project nature, such as stricter rules for children's drugs or finding sufficient patients for rare diseases [91].

Clinical trials challenges involving the same drugs were conducted simultaneously, causing concerns about redundancy and waste [92]. Therapeutic repurposing has potential, but many candidates fail clinical trials due to insufficient effectiveness or safety profiles [92]. Legal issues, such as limited patent coverage and hurdles during trials, also reduce the chance of success. Human clinical studies are costly and may not produce the intended return on investment [93].

We should use precision medicine strategies like patient stratification and biomarker-driven selection to identify cancer drug repurposing subpopulations and benefit from drug repurposing. Use innovative clinical trial methodologies, such as adaptive designs and master protocols, to efficiently analyze many repurposed medication combinations.

5.3 Predictive bioinformatics tools for drug repurposing requires confirmation

Predictive bioinformatics tools for cancer drug repurposing face challenges such as accuracy, biological complexity, and insufficient experimental validation [31]. Complex algorithms and heterogeneous datasets can lead to unreliable results, while tumor heterogeneity and resistance mechanisms complicate the modeling process [94]. Insufficient experimental validation requires significant resources and time. Prioritizing experimental validation and integrating advanced methodologies, such as HTS and machine learning, will further improve reliability and clinical relevance to confirm efficacy and improve translational potential in repurposed cancer therapies [95].

5.4 Intellectual property barriers and profit concern

The literature identifies hurdles to medication repurposing in the pharmaceutical business, such as patenting various chemicals, which prevents others from creating without a license. Limited patent time for failed compounds and limited return on investment are problems of repurposed drugs [96]. Collaborative partnerships among academia, pharmaceutical companies, and non-profit organizations can help address challenges in intellectual property rights negotiation, improve access to compounds for repurposing, and incentivize research into new uses for existing drugs through patent pools and open licensing models [97].

Drug repurposing faces challenges due to financial barriers, despite its potential benefits, resulting in slow uptake [98]. Organizations need financial resources and expertise to advance drug candidates [32]. Because pharmaceutical research and development frequently focusses on certain therapeutic areas inside an organization, making it challenging to recognize the potential of molecules to be repurposed outside this emphasis [99]. Limited return on investment discourages industries from funding trials. As such, multi-partner cooperation in repurposing is frequently required [100].

5.5 Biases affecting drug repurposing

Drug repurposing is typically the result of retrospective studies, which can be susceptible to time to death bias and selection bias [101]. Continuous research, which follow patients through lifelong therapy, might be particularly subject to eternal time bias, resulting in the fabrication of treatment benefits [102]. Most of the research on metformin and cancer incidence has demonstrated bias, raising doubts about the reliability of studies aimed at discovering novel candidates for repurposing. Drugs tested initially for their original indication usually target groups that are non-healthy, leading to selection biases. For instance, metformin's cohort studies used patients with diabetes, causing a selection bias [103]. This underscores the necessity for a more organized methodology in target identification that incorporates previously discussed techniques [101]. To mitigate biases in drug repurposing for cancer, diverse datasets, including multi-omics data from preclinical models, patient samples, and real-world evidence, are crucial. Additionally, reducing publication bias and promoting inconclusive results are essential (**Figure 3**) [104].

5.6 Knowledge access barrier

Obstacles to obtaining shelved compounds and their associated trial data present significant challenges in drug repurposing [105]. Often, compounds that are abandoned become inaccessible, with trial data remaining unpublished or concealed as trade secrets [106]. Gaining access to these compounds typically requires an internal advocate within the company, which is complicated by the company's reluctance to share potentially valuable compounds with competitors [107]. In contrast, non-profits and government-funded organizations face fewer commercial constraints. Additionally, the lack of repositories for abandoned drugs and the difficulty of digitizing paper records contribute to the problem. As experts leave and teams are disbanded, institutional knowledge about these compounds is lost. Mining and integrating large datasets also present significant logistical and technical challenges [108]. To improve cancer drug repurposing, centralized repositories, data-sharing agreements,

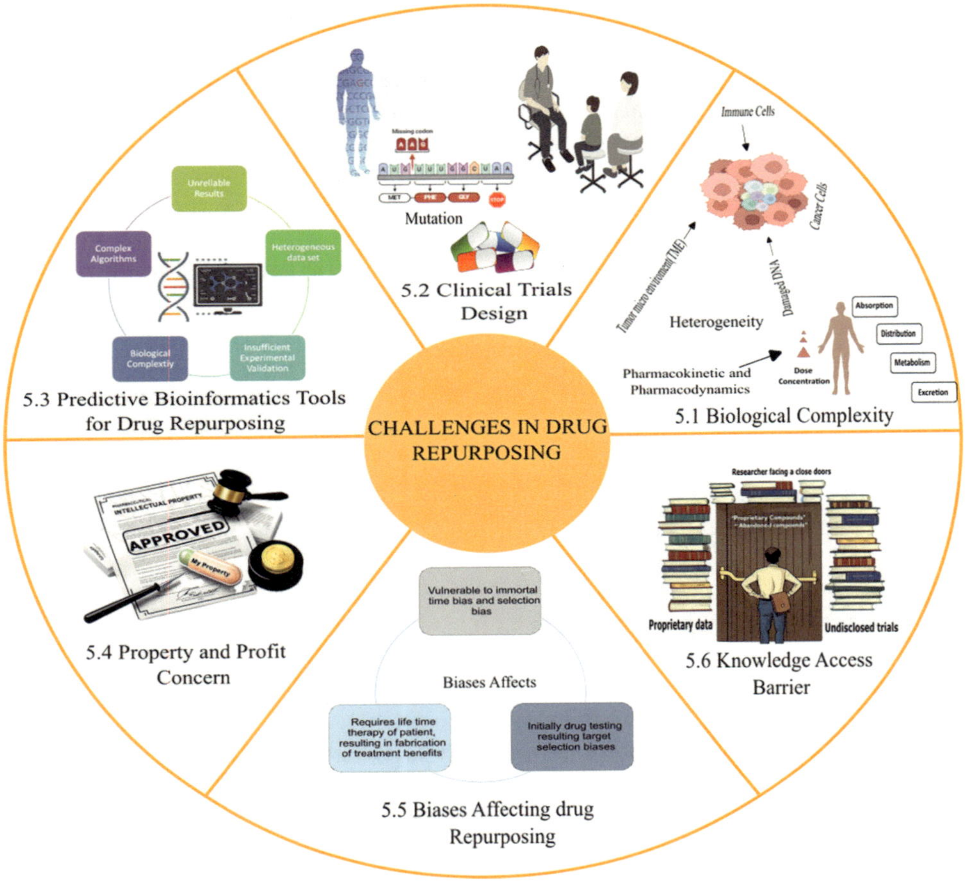

Figure 3.
Representation of challenges in drugs repurposing. (5.1) Describe the complexity of cancer cell by highlighting the heterogeneity, TME, pharmacodynamic and pharmacokinetic issues. (5.2) Illustrate the genetic mutation and diversity of cancer patient population. (5.3) Subsequent challenges occur while using predictive bioinformatics tools for cancer drug repurposing. (5.4) Patenting hurdles and profitability concerns. (5.5) Demonstrate the selection biases of target and time biases of repurposed drug. (5.6) Researchers often face barriers like limited funding, restricted access to data.

and advanced data mining techniques are needed to promote transparency, facilitate collaboration, and efficiently manage large datasets, thereby enhancing data accessibility. Promoting trial digitization and supporting regulatory policies that require clinical trial data disclosure can help decrease barriers.

5.7 Artificial intelligence in drug repurposing

AI is transforming drug repurposing by identifying new therapeutic targets, predicting drug-target interactions, and performing virtual screenings. AI can discover new uses for approved drugs by analyzing off-target effects and combining data from various sources, potentially speeding up treatment development for a variety of diseases. However, challenges remain, such as the need for high-quality datasets, interpretability issues, and potential biases in training data. High computational requirements and experimental validation are also obstacles, highlighting the importance of carefully integrating AI into drug repurposing efforts [109, 110].

6. Conclusion

Drug repurposing offers a cost-effective and time-efficient alternative to traditional drug development, which can take decades and involve high costs. By using existing drugs with known safety profiles, repurposing expedites the process of finding new treatments, particularly for cancer. This strategy has proven successful in various cases, such as thalidomide for multiple myeloma and metformin for BC. However, significant challenges remain, including biological complexity, clinical trial design, and intellectual property barriers. The heterogeneity of cancer makes it difficult to find universally effective repurposed drugs. Moreover, clinical trials for repurposed drugs must navigate intricate regulatory frameworks, and companies may be reluctant to invest in repurposing due to lower financial returns. AI is advancing drug repurposing by identifying new targets and accelerating development, though challenges like data quality and interpretability require careful integration. Overall, while repurposing of drug presents a promising approach to expanding cancer treatment options, addressing these challenges through collaboration, advanced bioinformatics tools, and better trial design will be crucial to unlocking its full potential.

Acknowledgements

The author acknowledges the use of AI tools for language and graphic polishing of the manuscript.

Author details

Rabia Zafar, Iqra Safdar, Aaiza Munir, Maah Rukh Zahid and Saad Serfraz*
Evolutionary Biology Lab, CABB, University of Agriculture Faisalabad, Pakistan

*Address all correspondence to: saad.serfraz@uaf.edu.pk; serfraz.saad@gmail.com

References

[1] Kulkarni VS, Alagarsamy V, Solomon VR, Jose PA, Murugesan S. Drug repurposing: An effective tool in modern drug discovery. Russian Journal of Bioorganic Chemistry. 2023;**49**(2):157-166

[2] Xue H, Li J, Xie H, Wang Y. Review of drug repositioning approaches and resources. International Journal of Biological Sciences. 2018;**14**(10):1232

[3] Sertkaya A, Birkenbach A, Berlind A, Eyraud J. Examination of Clinical Trial Costs and Barriers for Drug Development. US Department of Health and Human Services. Assis Secret Plan Eval; 2014

[4] Zong N, Wen A, Moon S, Fu S, Wang L, Zhao Y, et al. Computational drug repurposing based on electronic health records: A scoping review. npj Digital Medicine. 2022;**5**(1):77

[5] Choudhari AS, Mandave PC, Deshpande M, Ranjekar P, Prakash O. Phytochemicals in cancer treatment: From preclinical studies to clinical practice. Frontiers in Pharmacology. 2020;**10**:1614

[6] Sung H, Ferlay J, Siegel RL, Laversanne M, Soerjomataram I, Jemal A, et al. Global cancer statistics 2020: GLOBOCAN estimates of incidence and mortality worldwide for 36 cancers in 185 countries. CA: a Cancer Journal for Clinicians. 2021;**71**(3):209-249

[7] Iqbal MJ, Javed Z, Herrera-Bravo J, Sadia H, Anum F, Raza S, et al. Biosensing chips for cancer diagnosis and treatment: A new wave towards clinical innovation. Cancer Cell International. 2022;**22**(1):354

[8] Schein CH. Repurposing approved drugs for cancer therapy. British Medical Bulletin. 2021;**137**(1):13-27

[9] Fu L, Jin W, Zhang J, Zhu L, Lu J, Zhen Y, et al. Repurposing non-oncology small-molecule drugs to improve cancer therapy: Current situation and future directions. Acta Pharmaceutica Sinica B. 2022;**12**(2):532-557

[10] Huang F, Zhang C, Liu Q, Zhao Y, Zhang Y, Qin Y, et al. Identification of amitriptyline HCl, flavin adenine dinucleotide, azacitidine and calcitriol as repurposing drugs for influenza A H5N1 virus-induced lung injury. PLoS Pathogens. 2020;**16**(3):e1008341

[11] Pushpakom S, Iorio F, Eyers PA, Escott KJ, Hopper S, Wells A, et al. Drug repurposing: Progress, challenges and recommendations. Nature Reviews Drug Discovery. 2019;**18**(1):41-58

[12] Zheng W, Thorne N, McKew JC. Phenotypic screens as a renewed approach for drug discovery. Drug Discovery Today. 2013;**18**(21-22):1067-1073

[13] Jin G, Wong STC. Toward better drug repositioning: Prioritizing and integrating existing methods into efficient pipelines. Drug Discovery Today. 2014;**19**(5):637-644

[14] Sloane DA, Trikic MZ, Chu MLH, Lamers MBAC, Mason CS, Mueller I, et al. Drug-resistant aurora A mutants for cellular target validation of the small molecule kinase inhibitors MLN8054 and MLN8237. ACS Chemical Biology. 2010;**5**(6):563-576

[15] Molina DM, Jafari R, Ignatushchenko M, Seki T, Larsson EA,

Dan C, et al. Monitoring drug target engagement in cells and tissues using the cellular thermal shift assay. Science. 2013;**341**(6141):84-87

[16] Bago R, Sommer E, Castel P, Crafter C, Bailey FP, Shpiro N, et al. The hVps34-SGK 3 pathway alleviates sustained PI3K/Akt inhibition by stimulating mTORC 1 and tumour growth. The EMBO Journal. 2016;**35**(17):1902-1922

[17] Karaman MW, Herrgard S, Treiber DK, Gallant P, Atteridge CE, Campbell BT, et al. A quantitative analysis of kinase inhibitor selectivity. Nature Biotechnology. 2008;**26**(1):127-132

[18] Iljin K, Ketola K, Vainio P, Halonen P, Kohonen P, Fey V, et al. High-throughput cell-based screening of 4910 known drugs and drug-like small molecules identifies disulfiram as an inhibitor of prostate cancer cell growth. Clinical Cancer Research. 2009;**15**(19): 6070-6078

[19] Wu H, Huang J, Zhong Y, Huang Q. DrugSig: A resource for computational drug repositioning utilizing gene expression signatures. PLoS ONE. 2017;**12**(5):e0177743

[20] Iorio F, Rittman T, Ge H, Menden M, Saez-Rodriguez J. Transcriptional data: A new gateway to drug repositioning? Drug Discovery Today. 2013;**18**(7-8):350-357

[21] Dudley JT, Deshpande T, Butte AJ. Exploiting drug–disease relationships for computational drug repositioning. Briefings in Bioinformatics. 2011;**12**(4):303-311

[22] Park K. A review of computational drug repurposing. Translational and Clinical Pharmacology. 2019;**27**(2):59-63

[23] Pacini C, Iorio F, Gonçalves E, Iskar M, Klabunde T, Bork P, et al. DvD: An R/Cytoscape pipeline for drug repurposing using public repositories of gene expression data. Bioinformatics. 2013;**29**(1):132-134

[24] Troisi J, Cavallo P, Colucci A, Pierri L, Scala G, Symes S, et al. Metabolomics in genetic testing. Advances in Clinical Chemistry. 2020;**94**:85-153

[25] Pulley JM, Rhoads JP, Jerome RN, Challa AP, Erreger KB, Joly MM, et al. Using what we already have: Uncovering new drug repurposing strategies in existing omics data. Annual Review of Pharmacology and Toxicology. 2020;**60**(1):333-352

[26] Reddy AS, Zhang S. Polypharmacology: Drug discovery for the future. Expert Review of Clinical Pharmacology. 2013;**6**(1):41-47

[27] Issa NT, Peters OJ, Byers SW, Dakshanamurthy S. RepurposeVS: A drug repurposing-focused computational method for accurate drug-target signature predictions. Combinatorial Chemistry and High Throughput Screening. 2015;**18**(8):784-794

[28] Sekhon BS. Repositioning drugs and biologics: Retargeting old/existing drugs for potential new therapeutic applications. Journal of Pharmaceutical Education & Research. 2013;**4**(1):1

[29] Galvin BD, Li Z, Villemaine E, Poole CB, Chapman MS, Pollastri MP, et al. A target repurposing approach identifies N-myristoyltransferase as a new candidate drug target in filarial nematodes. PLoS Neglected Tropical Diseases. 2014;**8**(9):e3145

[30] Fogel DB. Factors associated with clinical trials that fail and opportunities

for improving the likelihood of success: A review. Contemporary Clinical Trials Communications. 2018;**11**:156-164

[31] Xia Y, Sun M, Huang H, Jin WL. Drug repurposing for cancer therapy. Signal Transduction and Targeted Therapy. 2024;**9**(1):92

[32] Novac N. Challenges and opportunities of drug repositioning. Trends in Pharmacological Sciences. 2013;**34**(5):267-272

[33] Young LY, Koda-Kimble MA. Applied Therapeutics: The Clinical Use of Drugs. 6th ed. Vancouver, WA: Applied Therapeutics, Inc.; 1995. DOI: 10.1604/9780915486236 1995

[34] Block SG, Nemeroff CB. Emerging antidepressants to treat major depressive disorder. Asian Journal of Psychiatry. 2014;**12**:7-16

[35] Latif T, Chauhan N, Khan R, Moran A, Usmani SZ. Thalidomide and its analogues in the treatment of multiple myeloma. Experimental Hematology & Oncology. 2012;**1**:1-8

[36] Sankaranarayanan R, Kumar DR, Altinoz MA, Bhat GJ. Mechanisms of colorectal cancer prevention by aspirin—A literature review and perspective on the role of COX-dependent and-independent pathways. International Journal of Molecular Sciences. 2020;**21**(23):9018

[37] Kim DJ, Kim J, Spaunhurst K, Montoya J, Khodosh R, Chandra K, et al. Open-label, exploratory phase II trial of oral itraconazole for the treatment of basal cell carcinoma. Journal of Clinical Oncology. 2014;**32**(8):745-751

[38] Pasquier E, André N, Street J, Chougule A, Rekhi B, Ghosh J, et al. Effective management of advanced angiosarcoma by the synergistic combination of propranolol and vinblastine-based metronomic chemotherapy: A bench to bedside study. eBioMedicine. 2016;**6**:87-95

[39] Hua Y, Zheng Y, Yao Y, Jia R, Ge S, Zhuang A. Metformin and cancer hallmarks: Shedding new lights on therapeutic repurposing. Journal of Translational Medicine. 2023;**21**(1):403

[40] Vazquez-Martin A, Oliveras-Ferraros C, Menendez JA. The antidiabetic drug metformin suppresses HER2 (erbB-2) oncoprotein overexpression via inhibition of the mTOR effector p70S6K1 in human breast carcinoma cells. Cell Cycle. 2009;**8**(1):88-96

[41] Memmott RM, Mercado JR, Maier CR, Kawabata S, Fox SD, Dennis PA. Metformin prevents tobacco carcinogen–induced lung tumorigenesis. Cancer Prevention Research. 2010;**3**(9):1066-1076

[42] Viollet B, Guigas B, Garcia NS, Leclerc J, Foretz M, Andreelli F. Cellular and molecular mechanisms of metformin: An overview. Clinical Science. 2012;**122**(6):253-270

[43] Boshuizen J, Peeper DS. Rational cancer treatment combinations: An urgent clinical need. Molecular Cell. 2020;**78**(6):1002-1018

[44] Guerini AE, Triggiani L, Maddalo M, Bonù ML, Frassine F, Baiguini A, et al. Mebendazole as a candidate for drug repurposing in oncology: An extensive review of current literature. Cancers. 2019;**11**(9):1284

[45] Bai RY, Staedtke V, Aprhys CM, Gallia GL, Riggins GJ. Antiparasitic mebendazole shows survival benefit in 2 preclinical models of glioblastoma

multiforme. Neuro-Oncology. 2011;**13**(9):974-982

[46] Mohi-Ud-Din R, Chawla A, Sharma P, Mir PA, Potoo FH, Reiner Ž, et al. Repurposing approved non-oncology drugs for cancer therapy: A comprehensive review of mechanisms, efficacy, and clinical prospects. European Journal of Medical Research. 2023;**28**(1):345

[47] Garg M, Kanojia D, Mayakonda A, Ganesan TS, Sadhanandhan B, Suresh S, et al. Selinexor (KPT-330) has antitumor activity against anaplastic thyroid carcinoma in vitro and in vivo and enhances sensitivity to doxorubicin. Scientific Reports. 2017;**7**(1):9749

[48] Motawi TMK, Sadik NAH, Fahim SA, Shouman SA. Combination of imatinib and clotrimazole enhances cell growth inhibition in T47D breast cancer cells. Chemico-Biological Interactions. 2015;**233**:147-156

[49] Kesh K, Gupta VK, Durden B, Garrido V, Mateo-Victoriano B, Lavania SP, et al. Therapy resistance, cancer stem cells and ECM in cancer: The matrix reloaded. Cancers. 2020;**12**(10):3067

[50] Weth FR, Hoggarth GB, Weth AF, Paterson E, White MPJ, Tan ST, et al. Unlocking hidden potential: Advancements, approaches, and obstacles in repurposing drugs for cancer therapy. British Journal of Cancer. 2024;**130**(5):703-715

[51] Malla R, Viswanathan S, Makena S, Kapoor S, Verma D, Raju AA, et al. Revitalizing cancer treatment: Exploring the role of drug repurposing. Cancers. 2024;**16**(8):1463

[52] Stuelten CH, Parent CA, Montell DJ. Cell motility in cancer invasion and metastasis: Insights from simple model organisms. Nature Reviews Cancer. 2018;**18**(5):296-312

[53] Joe NS, Godet I, Milki N, Ain NUI, Oza HH, Riggins GJ, et al. Mebendazole prevents distant organ metastases in part by decreasing ITGβ4 expression and cancer stemness. Breast Cancer Research. 2022;**24**(1):98

[54] Zhang J, Wei W, Zhong Q, Feng K, Yang R, Jiang Q. Budding uninhibited by benzimidazoles 1 promotes cell proliferation, invasion, and epithelial-mesenchymal transition via the Wnt/β-catenin signaling in glioblastoma. Heliyon. 2023;**9**(6):16996. DOI: 10.1016/j.heliyon.2023.e16996

[55] Sainero-Alcolado L, Liaño-Pons J, Ruiz-Pérez MV, Arsenian-Henriksson M. Targeting mitochondrial metabolism for precision medicine in cancer. Cell Death and Differentiation. 2022;**29**(7):1304-1317

[56] Wang J, Wu K, Bai F, Zhai H, Xie H, Du Y, et al. Celecoxib could reverse the hypoxia-induced Angiopoietin-2 upregulation in gastric cancer. Cancer Letters. 2006;**242**(1):20-27

[57] Schreiber RD, Old LJ, Smyth MJ. Cancer immunoediting: Integrating immunity's roles in cancer suppression and promotion. Science. 2011;**331**(6024):1565-1570

[58] Pertino MW, Vega C, Rolón M, Coronel C, Rojas de Arias A, Schmeda-Hirschmann G. Antiprotozoal activity of triazole derivatives of dehydroabietic acid and oleanolic acid. Molecules. 2017;**22**(3):369

[59] Xu QF, Peng HP, Lu XR, Hu Y, Xu ZH, Xu JK. Oleanolic acid regulates the Treg/Th17 imbalance in gastric

cancer by targeting IL-6 with miR-98-5p. Cytokine. 2021;**148**:155656

[60] Roder C, Thomson MJ. Auranofin: Repurposing an old drug for a golden new age. Drugs in R&D. 2015;**15**:13-20

[61] Chopra S, Goda JS, Mittal P, Mulani J, Pant S, Pai V, et al. Concurrent chemoradiation and brachytherapy alone or in combination with nelfinavir in locally advanced cervical cancer (NELCER): Study protocol for a phase III trial. BMJ Open. 2022;**12**(4):e055765

[62] Zheng C, Yan S, Lu L, Yao H, He G, Chen S, et al. Lovastatin inhibits EMT and metastasis of triple-negative breast cancer stem cells through dysregulation of cytoskeleton-associated proteins. Frontiers in Oncology. 2021;**11**: 656687

[63] Lin Y, Wang H, Tsai M, Su Y, Yang M, Chien C. Angiotensin II receptor blockers valsartan and losartan improve survival rate clinically and suppress tumor growth via apoptosis related to PI3K/AKT signaling in nasopharyngeal carcinoma. Cancer. 2021;**127**(10):1606-1619

[64] Aggarwal S, Verma SS, Aggarwal S, Gupta SC. Drug repurposing for breast cancer therapy: Old weapon for new battle. In: Seminars in cancer Biology. Vol. 68. Academic Press; 2021. pp. 8-20. DOI: 10.1016/j.semcancer.2019.09.012

[65] Qiao X, Wang X, Shang Y, Li Y, Chen S-Z. Azithromycin enhances anticancer activity of TRAIL by inhibiting autophagy and up-regulating the protein levels of DR4/5 in colon cancer cells in vitro and in vivo. Cancer Communications. 2018;**38**:1-13

[66] Li F, Huang J, Ji D, Meng Q, Wang C, Chen S, et al. Azithromycin effectively inhibits tumor angiogenesis by suppressing vascular endothelial growth factor receptor 2-mediated signaling pathways in lung cancer. Oncology Letters. 2017;**14**(1):89-96

[67] Liu Q, Zhou X, Li C, Zhang X, Li CL. Rapamycin promotes the anticancer action of dihydroartemisinin in breast cancer MDA-MB-231 cells by regulating expression of Atg7 and DAPK. Oncology Letters. 2018;**15**(4):5781-5786

[68] Gurova KV, Hill JE, Guo C, Prokvolit A, Burdelya LG, Samoylova E, et al. Small molecules that reactivate p53 in renal cell carcinoma reveal a NF-κB-dependent mechanism of p53 suppression in tumors. National Academy of Sciences of the United States of America. 2005;**102**(48):17448-17453

[69] Gupta N, Gaikwad S, Kaushik I, Wright SE, Markiewski MM, Srivastava SK. Atovaquone suppresses triple-negative breast tumor growth by reducing immune-suppressive cells. International Journal of Molecular Sciences. 2021;**22**(10):5150

[70] Zhao Y, Cao J, Melamed A, Worley M, Gockley A, Jones D, et al. Losartan treatment enhances chemotherapy efficacy and reduces ascites in ovarian cancer models by normalizing the tumor stroma. National Academy of Sciences of the United States of America. 2019;**116**(6):2210-2219

[71] Yao H, Jiang L, Lin X, Liang ZG. Fluvastatin combined with benazepril may contribute to the favorable prognosis of patients with atrial fibrillation. Biomedicine and Pharmacotherapy. 2016;**83**:687-692

[72] de Souza CO, Kurauti MA, de Fatima SF, de Morais H, Curi R, Hirabara SM, et al. Celecoxib and ibuprofen restore the ATP content and the gluconeogenesis activity in the

liver of walker-256 tumor-bearing rats. Cellular Physiology and Biochemistry. 2015;**36**(4):1659-1669

[73] Li Y, Acharya G, Elahy M, Xin H, Khachigian LM. The anthelmintic flubendazole blocks human melanoma growth and metastasis and suppresses programmed cell death protein-1 and myeloid-derived suppressor cell accumulation. Cancer Letters. 2019;**459**:268-276

[74] Samy ALPA, Bakthavachalam V, Vudutha M, Vinjamuri S, Chinnapaka S, Munirathinam G. Eprinomectin, a novel semi-synthetic macrocylic lactone is cytotoxic to PC3 metastatic prostate cancer cells via inducing apoptosis. Toxicology and Applied Pharmacology. 2020;**401**:115071

[75] Verhees F, Legemaate D, Demers I, Jacobs R, Haakma WE, Rousch M, et al. The antiviral agent cidofovir induces DNA damage and mitotic catastrophe in HPV-positive and-negative head and neck squamous cell carcinomas in vitro. Cancers. 2019;**11**(7):919

[76] Tan H, He L, Cheng Z. Inhibition of eIF4E signaling by ribavirin selectively targets lung cancer and angiogenesis. Biochemical and Biophysical Research Communications. 2020;**529**(3):519-525

[77] Iwasaki H, Inoue H, Mitsuke Y, Badran A, Ikegaya S, Ueda T. Doxycycline induces apoptosis by way of caspase-3 activation with inhibition of matrix metalloproteinase in human T-lymphoblastic leukemia CCRF-CEM cells. The Journal of Laboratory and Clinical Medicine. 2002;**140**(6):382-386

[78] Ho Y, Duh J, Jeng J, Wang Y, Liang Y, Lin C, et al. Griseofulvin potentiates antitumorigenesis effects of nocodazole through induction of apoptosis and G2/M cell cycle arrest in human colorectal cancer cells. International Journal of Cancer. 2001;**91**(3):393-401

[79] Pan JX, Ding K, Wang CY. Niclosamide, an old antihelminthic agent, demonstrates antitumor activity by blocking multiple signaling pathways of cancer stem cells. Chinese Journal of Cancer. 2012;**31**(4):178

[80] Colafigli M, Ciccullo A, Borghetti A, Fanti I, Melis F, Modica S, et al. Impact of antiretroviral therapy on the risk of recurrence in HIV-1 infected patients with Kaposi sarcoma: A multicenter cohort experience. Journal of Clinical Medicine. 2019;**8**(12):2062

[81] Chen YX, Gao QY, Zou TH, Wang BM, Liu SD, Sheng JQ, et al. Berberine versus placebo for the prevention of recurrence of colorectal adenoma: A multicentre, double-blinded, randomised controlled study. The Lancet Gastroenterology and Hepatology. 2020;**5**(3):267-275

[82] Danjuma MI, Entonu ME, Emmanuel E. Drug repurposing: Recent advancements, challenges, and future therapeutics for cancer treatment. Journal of Bacteriology & Mycology: Open Access. 2022;**10**(2):26-30

[83] Grizzi F, Chiriva-Internati M. Cancer: Looking for simplicity and finding complexity. Cancer Cell International. 2006;**6**(1):4. DOI: 10.1186/1475-2867-6-4

[84] Brafford P, Herlyn M. Gene expression profiling of melanoma cells–searching the haystack. Journal of Translational Medicine. 2005;**3**:1-2

[85] Proietto M, Crippa M, Damiani C, Pasquale V, Sacco E, Vanoni M, et al. Tumor heterogeneity: Preclinical models, emerging technologies, and future

applications. Frontiers in Oncology. 2023;**13**:1164535. DOI: 10.3389/fonc.2023.1164535

[86] Zhu L, Jiang M, Wang H, Sun H, Zhu J, Zhao W, et al. A narrative review of tumor heterogeneity and challenges to tumor drug therapy. Annals of Translational Medicine. 2021;**9**(16):1351-1351. DOI: 10.21037/atm-21-1948

[87] Zhu X, Liang R, Lan T, Ding D, Huang S, Shao J, et al. Tumor-associated macrophage-specific CD155 contributes to M2-phenotype transition, immunosuppression, and tumor progression in colorectal cancer. The Journal for ImmunoTherapy of Cancer. 2022;**10**(9):e004219. Available from: http://jitc.bmj.com/content/10/9/e004219.abstract

[88] Tan HW, Seen DLT, Xu YM, Lau ATY. Cadmium, cellular senescence, and cancer. Reviews of Environmental Contamination and Toxicology. 2023;**261**(1):21. DOI: 10.1007/s44169-023-00042-0

[89] Alarcon-Barrera JC, Kostidis S, Ondo-Mendez A, Giera M. Recent advances in metabolomics analysis for early drug development. Drug Discovery Today. 2022;**27**(6):1763-1773

[90] Flemming A. Unleashing NK cell anti-metastatic activity. Nature Reviews Drug Discovery. 2014;**13**(4):257

[91] Roessler HI, Knoers NVAM, van Haelst MM, van Haaften G. Drug repurposing for rare diseases. Trends in Pharmacological Sciences. 2021;**42**(4):255-267. DOI: 10.1016/j.tips.2021.01.003

[92] Lynch HF, Caplan A, Furlong P, Bateman-House A. Helpful lessons and cautionary tales: How should COVID-19 drug development and access inform approaches to non-pandemic diseases? The American Journal of Bioethics. 2021;**21**(12):4-19

[93] Parisi D, Adasme MF, Sveshnikova A, Bolz SN, Moreau Y, Schroeder M. Drug repositioning or target repositioning: A structural perspective of drug-target-indication relationship for available repurposed drugs. Computational and Structural Biotechnology Journal. 2020;**18**:1043-1055

[94] Hernández-Lemus E, Martínez-García M. Pathway-based drug-repurposing schemes in cancer: The role of translational bioinformatics. Frontiers in Oncology. 2021;**10**:605680

[95] Zhou H, Liu H, Yu Y, Yuan X, Xiao L. Informatics on drug repurposing for breast cancer. Drug Design, Development and Therapy. 2023;**17**:1933-1943

[96] Doshi S, Chepuri SP. A computational approach to drug repurposing using graph neural networks. Computers in Biology and Medicine. 2022;**150**:105992

[97] Hernandez JJ, Pryszlak M, Smith L, Yanchus C, Kurji N, Shahani VM, et al. Giving drugs a second chance: Overcoming regulatory and financial hurdles in repurposing approved drugs as cancer therapeutics. Frontiers in Oncology. 2017;7:273

[98] Halabi SF. The drug repurposing ecosystem: Intellectual property incentives, market exclusivity, and the future of new medicines. Yale Journal of Law & Technology. 2018;**20**:1

[99] Tartaglia LA. Complementary new approaches enable repositioning of failed drug candidates. Expert Opinion on Investigational Drugs. 2006;**15**(11):1295-1298

[100] Cha Y, Erez T, Reynolds IJ, Kumar D, Ross J, Koytiger G, et al. Drug

repurposing from the perspective of pharmaceutical companies. British Journal of Pharmacology. 2018;**175**(2):168-180

[101] Tran AA, Prasad V. Drug repurposing for cancer treatments: A well-intentioned, but misguided strategy. The Lancet Oncology. 2020;**21**(9):1134-1136

[102] Tyrer F, Bhaskaran K, Rutherford MJ. Immortal time bias for life-long conditions in retrospective observational studies using electronic health records. BMC Medical Research Methodology. 2022;**22**(1):86

[103] Suissa S, Azoulay L. Metformin and the risk of cancer: Time-related biases in observational studies. Diabetes Care. 2012;**35**(12):2665-2673

[104] Hwang TJ, Franklin JM, Chen CT, Lauffenburger JC, Gyawali B, Kesselheim AS, et al. Efficacy, safety, and regulatory approval of Food and Drug Administration–designated breakthrough and nonbreakthrough cancer medicines. Journal of Clinical Oncology. 2018;**36**(18):1805-1812

[105] Nosengo N. Can you teach old drugs new tricks? Nature. 2016;**534**(7607):314-316

[106] Mandrioli R, Mercolini L. Discontinued anxiolytic drugs (2009-2014). Expert Opinion on Investigational Drugs. 2015;**24**(4):557-573

[107] Rogawski MA, Federoff HJ. Disclosure of clinical trial results when product development is abandoned. Science Translational Medicine. 2011;**3**(102):102cm29

[108] Krishnamurthy N, Grimshaw AA, Axson SA, Choe SH, Miller JE. Drug repurposing: A systematic review on root causes, barriers and facilitators. BMC Health Services Research. 2022;**22**(1):970. DOI: 10.1186/s12913-022-08272-z

[109] Quazi S. Role of artificial intelligence and machine learning in bioinformatics: Drug discovery and drug repurposing. Life Sciences. 2021. DOI: 10.20944/preprints202105.0346.v1

[110] Tanoli Z, Vähä-Koskela M, Aittokallio T. Artificial intelligence, machine learning, and drug repurposing in cancer. Expert Opinion on Drug Discovery. 2021;**16**(9):977-989

Chapter 5

Computational Drug Repositioning Method Applied to Lung Cancer

Sulekha Khute, Kareti Srinivasa Rao and Paranthaman Subash

Abstract

Lung cancer is the most common cancer affecting men and women worldwide. Among different types of lung cancer (LC), two primary forms stand out: small-cell lung cancer (SCLC) and non-small-cell lung cancer (NSCLC). NSCLC, the more prevalent variety, accounts for around 85–90% of all lung cancer cases. Drug repurposing, also known as drug repositioning, is the investigation of using existing drugs for new therapeutic purposes. This approach can lead to the formulation of effective treatments for diseases that might not have been adequately addressed by traditional drug discovery methods. The importance of drug repositioning in lung cancer research cannot be overstated. Traditional drug discovery is often a lengthy and costly process, requiring years of research and substantial investment. In contrast, repurposing existing medications can enhance the pre-clinical journey of developing new drugs. High-performance computing capabilities enable the efficient processing of these extensive datasets, which may include biological, biomedical, and electronic health-related information. This data-driven approach has dramatically accelerated the development of computational methods for drug repositioning. The strategy of drug repositioning offers a promising pathway for researchers, significantly shortening the timeline and reducing the costs associated with new drug development.

Keywords: lung cancer, ligand, drug repositioning, targets, in silico

1. Introduction

Over 1.3 million instances of lung cancer (LC) are reported each year, making it one of the most prevalent and deadliest cancer-related deaths globally [1]. LC is a largely incurable illness. LC is responsible for 25% of cancer-related fatalities and 14% of new cancer cases worldwide [1, 2]. LC claims more lives in the United States than the combined fatality toll from the other four primary forms of cancer. Two types of LCs are there, which is illustrated in **Figure 1**. LC is very varied and may grow in several places along the bronchial tree, which can result in a broad range of symptoms [3]. Survival chances for LC may be increased by early identification via screening programs like low-dose CT scans. There are two types of lung cancer: SCLC, which is more difficult to treat than NSCLC [3]. Immunotherapy, radiation therapy, chemotherapy, targeted therapy, and surgery are among the available treatment options. 85% of LC cases are NSCLC, which may include subtypes such as giant cell carcinoma, squamous cell carcinoma, and adenocarcinoma [4].

IntechOpen

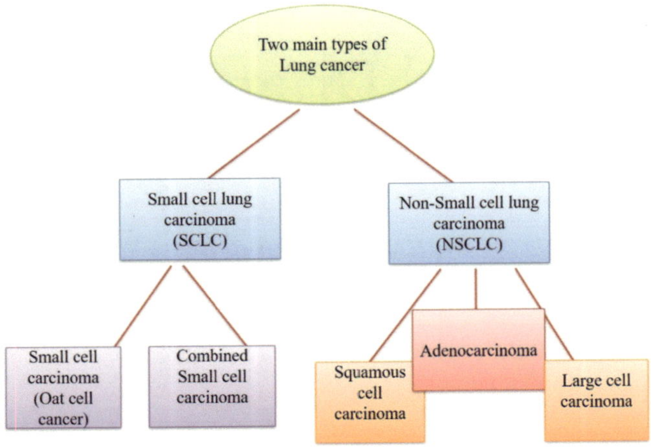

Figure 1.
Types of lung cancer.

NSCLC, or non-small-cell lung cancer, is a prevalent subtype seen in the outer lungs, with adenocarcinoma being the most common. Squamous cell carcinoma, an uncommon and aggressive form, is found in the bronchial tube lining. SCLS, a deadly, aggressive variety, accounts for 10–15% of all cases and is commonly detected at an advanced stage, making therapy problematic and resulting in reduced survival rates [5]. Early identification and individualized treatment methods are critical for improving results. The National Cancer Institute has devised numerous ways for detecting and diagnosing LC stages, with treatment choices differing depending on the patient's stage, susceptibility, health status, and molecular profile. The most effective medications for LC are still platinum-based chemotherapeutics like cisplatin, which are usually used in combination with other treatments, despite advancements in diagnostic technology and innovative chemotherapeutics [6].

Immunotherapy is a potential therapeutic option for LC, particularly in advanced instances. Targeted medicines targeting certain genetic mutations have shown promise in improving results. For non-small-cell lung cancer, cisplatin and other platinum-core medications are the first line of therapy. Premetrexed, gemcitabine, docetaxel, and paclitaxel are other chemotherapeutic agents [7–9]. Tyrosine kinase inhibitors (TKIs) are approved as first-line therapy for genetically alterations-related LC [10]. If first-line drugs fail, second-line therapies, including GCB, DTX, and pemetrexed, are commonly utilized [11]. Immunotherapy drugs including pembrolizumab and nivolumab have exhibited promise in treating non-small-cell LC, with individualized treatment options advised for patients with particular genetic abnormalities. Despite breakthroughs in cancer biology and innovative therapies, overall survival rates remain dismal [12, 13]. Treatments for LC are connected to a delayed development process, excessive price, regulatory obstacles, and high failure rates [13, 14]. Collaboration between academics and pharmaceutical corporations is vital for generating more effective and accessible therapies. A new drug generally takes 13 years and costs $1.8 billion to create [15].

The pharmaceutical industry and research have showed a strong interest in the process of drug repositioning. This is mostly due to its ability to discover fresh applications for already authorized pharmaceuticals and to accelerate the development of new ones. Drug repositioning is a preferable alternative to standard *de novo* drug development strategies because it is more time and cost efficient [16, 17]. Repositioning, also known as drug repurposing, drug reprofiling, drug redirection, drug retasking, or therapeutic switching, is the process of discovering new applications for already approved medications. The global coronavirus illness (COVID-19) pandemic, which started in China, has made the pharmaceutical repositioning strategy increasingly crucial. The rapid emergence of the pandemic and its capacity to spread to a significant number of individuals (with a reproduction number R0 larger

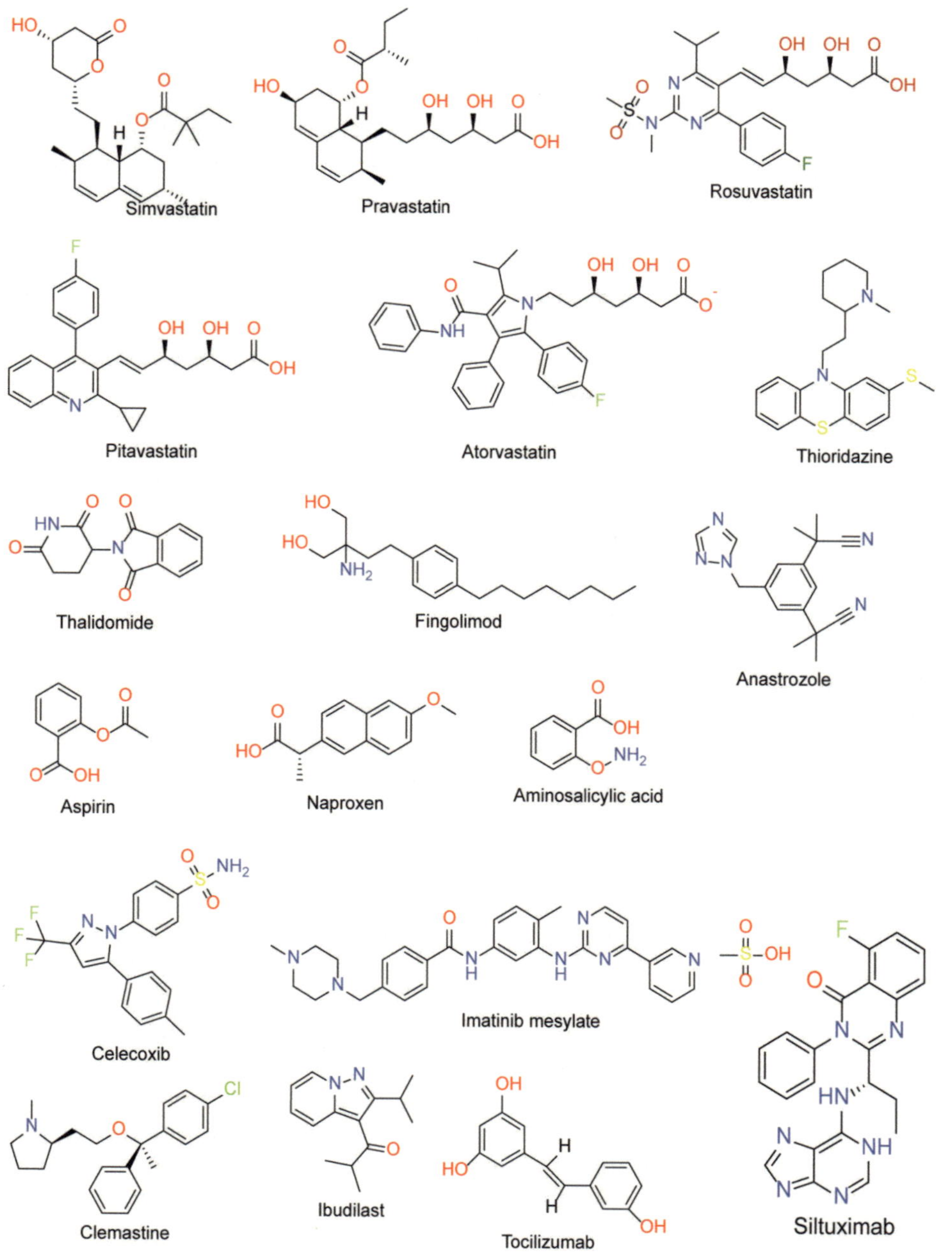

Figure 2.
Chemical structures of the drug to be repurposed for LC.

than 1 in the absence of social distance and other preventive measures) have created a pressing need to discover novel medications to address this illness. The progress of medication and vaccine research for COVID-19 is constantly evolving, with frequent updates on the current state of these efforts [18]. Traditional drug development is hindered by its sluggish pace, which is not suitable for the urgent need to create novel therapies and treatments. As a result, the quicker repositioning strategy has gained significant attention owing to its potential to identify compounds that may effectively address the consequences of viral infections [19–21].

In general, typical drug repositioning studies seek to discover parallels between medication effects and modes of action (MoA) [22]. These studies also seek to discover new applications for current medications by screening them against novel targets [23]. They consider common characteristics, such as adverse effects and chemical structures, across pharmaceutical compounds [24]. In addition, they search for links between drugs and ailments [25]. High-performance computers and the rapid accumulation of vast volumes of biological and electronic health data, such as publicly accessible databases, online health communities, and microarray gene expression profiles, have made it simpler to move pharmaceuticals around in computers. These techniques usually include network analysis, data mining, and machine learning [26]. An essential component of modern medication repositioning research is examining the correlation between various biological entities. The biological entities include several elements, such as medications, illnesses, genes, and adverse drug reactions (ADRs), among others. Chemical structures of the drug to be repurposed for LC are illustrated in **Figure 2**.

2. Drug repositioning strategies

The basics of drug repositioning are essentially twofold. First, since many diseases are linked, drugs used to treat one ailment may have an effect on others. Second, since medicines are inherently misleading, they may be related to a wide range of targets and pathways [27]. Thus, drug repositioning research may be classified into two types depending on the data source: (i) drug-based strategies, in which the discovery is based on drug-related data, and (ii) disease-based strategies, in which the discovery is based on information regarding illnesses.

3. Drug-based strategies

Drug-based approaches rely on drug-related data as the basis for forecasting therapeutic potentials and new uses for pharmaceuticals that have already received approval, including chemical, molecular, biological, pharmacological, and genetic data. When there is a great need to understand more about how pharmacological characteristics may affect drug repositioning or when a substantial quantity of drug-related data are available, drug-based techniques are used [28]. Most of the research in this category supports the premise that medication R2 is a good candidate to treat illness D if drug R1 is utilized to cure disease D, and both treatments have comparable profiles and modes of action. The two primary strategies that embody this category are the chemical structure and molecular information approach [29–31] and the genome strategy [32].

Drugs with comparable effects and mechanisms of action may be automatically identified utilizing the gene expression profile similarity developed by Iorio et al. [22].

The authors began by creating a drug network in which medicines are represented by nodes and edges demonstrate similarities between two drugs. Following that, they searched for drug communities using graph techniques. Drugs work similarly in all of these classes. As a result, Hu and Agarwal [33] explored drug variations in individuals and sickness gene expression using a negative correlation to build a disease-drug network that might predict potential uses for already-approved pharmaceuticals. Sirota et al. [34] identified fresh therapeutic repositioning opportunities by undertaking a thorough, systematic examination of gene expression patterns associated with a variety of disorders and treatments.

4. Disease-based strategies

Disease-based techniques rely on disease-related data, such as information on phenotypic features, side effects, and indications, to anticipate therapeutic potentials and innovative uses for already available medications. When there is a lack of drug-related data or when it is wanted to investigate how pharmacological elements may aid efforts to reposition drugs to target a certain sickness, disease-based strategies are used [25, 35, 36].

5. Phenome strategy

The phenome, defined as the entire set of phenotypic trait data, has emerged as a novel approach to linking medications with clinical outcomes for drug repositioning because it characterizes the physiological consequences of a drug's unintentional effects and biological activities. Furthermore, there may be a close relationship between the phenotypic presentation of a drug's side effects and the phenotypic manifestation of a disease, implying that the two illnesses may have same underlying processes [25].

According to research, unanticipated activities generated by pharmaceutical off-targets and clinical side effects might profile human phenotypic features, potentially leading to the identification of innovative therapeutic applications for these treatments in the future. Because there is a strong relationship between the binding patterns of targeted components and side-effect similarities, Campillos et al. [35] created a measure of side-effect similarity and experimentally demonstrated that it reveals potential therapeutic uses for already-approved drugs. According to Yang and Agarwal [37], clinical side effects may be exploited to construct a drug's phenotypic profile and identify new disease indications. To identify medication-disease correlations, a dataset on drug side effects was combined with a dataset on drug-disease connections. The next step was to construct a disease indicator prediction model using side effects as characteristics.

The premise upon which Ye et al.'s [38] drug-drug similarity network was built was that drugs with similar side effects would also have similar therapeutic uses. New medicinal indications were discovered beside the previously known ones. Using adverse effect data, Bisgin et al. [39] built a model to predict new therapeutic indications for existing drugs. It is important to note that using phenotypic characteristic data to forecast novel therapeutic indications requires a thorough understanding of molecular processes. While the majority of phenotypic-based research uses information from medication labels and clinical trials, Nugent et al. [40] analyzed social media side-effect data to find new therapeutic indications in addition to previously known indications.

Data on phenotypic features may be combined with information from other sources, such as the genome, to discover new uses for pharmaceuticals and treatment choices. Hoehndorf et al. [41] used phenotypic similarities to create genotype-disease correlations, which were then merged with genotype-disease relationship data to predict new drug-disease linkages. Using such a model, an integrated method for identifying drug-disease links for illnesses with no known biological etiology might be developed. Gottlieb et al. [42] created a model that uses a range of drug-drug similarity markers, such as phenome-based similarity, to predict novel drug-drug interactions and the severity associated with each. Drug-drug interactions, including a few surprising ones, were found by Sridhar et al. [36] using a range of drug-drug similarity criteria, such as phenotypic similarities with previously known drug-drug interactions.

5.1 Computational drug repositioning models: Validation

When compared to the conventional *de novo* drug discovery and development strategy, computational drug repositioning studies ideally save time and money by optimizing the pre-clinical stage of generating new treatments and finding new applications for previously approved medications. After validating and assessing their results, researchers offer a group of potential drugs for repositioning. Nevertheless, there is a chance that certain validation models will not be reliable and accurate or that validation/evaluation models will not match the suggested computational models in all circumstances. Therefore, understanding and selecting appropriate validation models are essential to the effectiveness of the computational models that have been suggested. Furthermore, because of a number of considerations, including high cost, high toxicity, low bioavailability, and the fact that certain pharmaceuticals have been discontinued or are not favored by doctors or biologists, choosing the appropriate group of drug repositioning candidates for validation is also essential. To advance the work being done in this area, it is crucial that all parties involved in the medication repositioning process be fully committed to it.

Practical validation and evaluation processes vary from study to study and may be dependent, at least in part, on the expected objectives. These models are classified into many areas, including electronic health data, leave-one-out and cross-validation, case studies, benchmarking against previous models, *in vitro* and *in vivo* trials, and interaction with domain experts. Despite numerous well-known limitations, *in vitro* and *in vivo* experiments have proven pharmaceutical repositioning prospects. *In vitro* and *in vivo* validation models refer to investigations that take place in a controlled environment without the use of a live creature (such as cellular biology studies conducted outside of organisms or cells) and in a whole living body (such as animal research and clinical trials), respectively. Albendazole was recognised by Lim et al. [43] as a pharmacological repositioning candidate with anti-cancer characteristics. In order to evaluate the potential efficacy of repositioned pharmaceuticals, Rakshit et al. [44] developed the On-Target Ratio (OTR), which is the ratio of the number of drug targets in their proposed disease-specific gene network to the total number of interactions with the same medication in the DrugBank database. Additionally, Ozsoy et al. [45] compared their results to those of ClinicalTrials.gov, a worldwide database of clinical studies funded by both public and commercial sources. In addition, the authors compared their model to the most sophisticated models and performed a leave-one-out test.

The efficiency of the models was assessed using Yang and Zhao [46] cross-referencing model for medical literature, which is based on scientific publications from PubMed. In order to ensure the accuracy of their suggested model, the authors also spoke with medical specialists on their results. The physicians reported that the repositioning drug candidates found using the recommended method offered a substantial advantage in terms of screening and lowering the number of medications that might be utilized for the approved indications. Zeng et al. [47] validated their proposed deep learning model, which searches for probable drug-disease correlations, using two case studies and an electronic health record validation model. Notably, as literature mining methods have advanced, literature-based validation models have become more popular in recent research. Furthermore, K-fold cross-validation is often used in machine learning research to train models and correct excessively optimistic model performance forecasts. This problem may potentially be resolved if more testing data that differ from the training set are supplied.

5.2 A computational method for repurposing drugs

Many different kinds of drugs have been repurposed, and there are also many different ways to achieve so. The computational technique, also known as "in silico drug repurposing," comprises the collection and analysis of a wide range of data from several sources, mostly databases that include details on electronic health records (EHRs), chemical structure, gene expression, and proteomics [48]. This method uses a variety of approaches and data to find and investigate possible drugs for repurposing.

Network-based medication repurposing is the first computational approach method that makes use of genotyping technological advancements by employing genome-wide association studies (GWAS) to identify genetic variations that impact prevalent illnesses [49]. New targets that are shared by multiple disease phenotypes are uncovered by GWAS, albeit they may not be therapeutic. Researchers may find druggable genes upstream or downstream of the target gene by employing network-based approaches [50, 51]. Drugs that have been repurposed using this technique include iloperidone, an antipsychotic used to treat schizophrenia, to treat hypertension [52], and vismodegib, an inhibitor of the Hedgehog signaling pathway, to treat Gorlin syndrome [53]. One such example is the random walk propagation approach, which adds genes that are neighbors in a gene-gene or protein-protein network to the list of genes linked with illness. Medications like methotrexate for Crohn's disease, cisplatin for breast cancer, donepezil for Parkinson's disease, and gabapentin for anxiety disorders were given another lease of life by the application of this approach [54].

Profile-based medication repurposing is an additional computational approach alternative that involves comparing the profile of one medication with that of another drug, ailment, or clinical characteristic [55]. One example is comparing the expression profile linked to the disease with the differential gene expression in a cell or tissue before and after therapy [56, 57]. Assume, for example, that a medicine has been found to block the transcription of a specific gene associated to the causation of a disease. If so, the medicine has the power to reverse the sickness and ought to be investigated for a new usage [56, 57]. An alternative profile-based strategy that may identify unique drug-target correlations studies the chemical structures of various drugs [58]. Molecular docking, which compares multiple ligands to a receptor, may be used to achieve this. Utilizing a computer docking technique, it was revealed that the antiparasitic medication mebendazole has the structural potential to block vascular endothelial growth factor receptor 2 (VEGFR2) [59].

6. Pros and cons of repurposing drugs

Time and money are the two key benefits of medication repurposing in cancer treatment. Research has shown that the typical duration between the submission of an exploratory drug application and the first new drug application for innovative antineoplastics is 8.3 years, whereas for repurposed medications, it is between 3 and 4 years [60, 61]. Because the repurposed drug's pharmacokinetics and pharmacodynamics are already known, a phase I clinical trial may not always be necessary, leading to an improved timetable. Cost is an additional benefit of medication repurposing. A reused medicine costs $300 million to commercialize, whereas a fresh drug needs $2–3 billion to create [62].

However, there are drawbacks to repurposing pharmaceuticals. For instance, repurposing a proven drug for a novel purpose has a significant chance of failure since the new course may not work out as intended. Furthermore, in order to guarantee their safety in the new population, certain repurposed medications may go through comparable time- and money-consuming procedures to those of innovative treatments [62].

7. Failures in drug repositioning

Repositioning drugs is not always successful. In a phase III study for gastric cancer, bevacizumab, a kinase inhibitor that has been repurposed to treat several other cancers, failed to show effectiveness [63]. Sunitinib, a multi-kinase inhibitor, was approved to treat GISTs, pancreatic neuroendocrine tumors, and renal cell carcinomas, among other diseases [64]. However, clinical studies for colorectal, breast, prostate, and NSCLC were unsuccessful. Since generic kinase-targeting drugs, such as sunitinib, are not successful in treating all cancers, more targeted strategies are needed. Although the two drugs had previously been authorized for the treatment of depression and opioid addiction, respectively, the FDA rejected the combination of bupropion and naltrexone in February 2011 because of possible cardiovascular side effects. In obese people, this mixture seems to work in concert to control energy expenditure and appetite. Therefore, even if a medicine has been moved and complies with clinical safety standards, it may still have unfavorable side effects. It is important to consider a drug's initial usage while relocating it. For example, the required doses of cytotoxic chemotherapy may harm healthy cells; therefore, it may not be the ideal option for treating hypertension [65]. Public libraries and algorithms for identifying different medications or biological markers are becoming more and more available, yet obstacles in the form of data management and omics-data integration continue to exist. Therefore, biologists, physicians, and other scientists without a background in computing may easily use web-based technologies. Web-based resources facilitate the interpretation of disease processes by researchers and make it easier to target the pharmacological features of medications for new uses. For web-based technologies that have been thoroughly examined lately, drug-associated entities including side effects, mechanisms of action, and drug-target or drug-drug interactions capture important data [66]. In this work, we gathered a few instances of drugs that have been repurposed for LC (as shown in **Table 1**) and web-based tools (as shown in **Table 2**) and used data unique to LC using web-based tools to repurpose medications.

S. no	Drug	Original indication	Mechanism for LC	Refs.
1.	Albendazole	Anthelmintic	It has been found to inhibit the expression of HIF-1α and VEGF in NSCLC cells.	[67, 68]
2.	Atenolol	Antihypertensive	Anticancer activity in lung cancer cell lines A549 and H1299, most effective in inhibiting colony formation and cell death.	[69]
3.	Atorvastatin	Lowers cholesterol	Lung cancer treatment in patients with advanced NSCLC treated with PD-1 inhibitors.	[70, 71]
4.	Atovaquone	Treatment of Pneumonia and Malaria	Exhibits stronger anti-cancer effects due to its regulation of pyruvate, glutamine, and TCA cycle across immune cells in tumour microenvironment.	[70, 72]
5.	Celecoxib	Treat osteoarthritis and Menstrual symptoms.	Celecoxib induces apoptosis in lung cancer cells through caspase cascades and DNA fragmentation, with DR5 expression playing a significant role. Combination with celecoxib enhances apoptosis.	[73, 74]
6.	Indomethacin	Reduce fever, pain and stiffness.	Indomethacin affects polyamine metabolism in NSCLC cells, enhancing the effect of polyamine synthesis inhibitors like MDL72527 or SAM486, by downregulating MRP1 and inducing apoptosis.	[75–78]
7.	Itraconazole	Antifungal	Itraconazole, a drug that inhibits the hedgehog pathway and angiogenesis, has shown promising results in clinical trials for lung cancer treatment.	[79–81]
8.	Levamisole	Treat parasitic worm infections	Levamisole inhibits JNK activity in lung cancer, promoting DR4-independent apoptosis via TRAIL. It reduces cell growth, promotes cell cycle arrest, and enhances DR4-independent death.	[82, 83]
9.	Lopinavir	Antiretroviral	Lovidin/ritonavir, a dual protease inhibitor, induces genotoxic stress on lung cells, altering gene expression and activating the p53 DNA damage response, potentially acting as an anti-cancer agent.	[84]
10.	Lovastatin	Treat high blood cholesterol	Lovastatin effectively regulates cancer cell proliferation, apoptosis, and drug resistance, including lung cancer, by inhibiting cell proliferation, regulating signalling pathways, and sensitizing cells to ionizing radiation.	[85]
11.	Metformin	Antidiabetic	Metformin, a medication with potential antitumor effects in NSCLC has been extensively studied in clinical trials for its potential use in cancer treatment.	[86, 87]
12.	Mebendazole	Anthelmintic	Mebendazole induces apoptosis and inhibits migration in NSCLC by increasing p53 protein stability through STAT3 signalling downregulation, potentially treating NSCLC through the ROS-JAK2-STAT3 pathway.	[88, 89]

S. no	Drug	Original indication	Mechanism for LC	Refs.
13.	Minocycline	Treat bacterial infections	Minocycline has been found to inhibit cancer cell proliferation, including lung cancer cells, in vitro and in vivo. Its molecular mechanism of cytotoxicity in lung cancer cells is unclear. Minocycline's good penetration into lung tissues may accelerate protein degradation, providing a new cancer therapy mechanism.	[90, 91]
14.	Pioglitazone	Thiazolidinediones	Pioglitazone may inhibit lung cancer cell glycolysis, potentially influencing cancer pathogenesis by downregulating specific proteins and affecting the TGFβ pathway, potentially affecting EMT and metastasis spread.	[92]
15.	Pitavastatin	Blood cholesterol lowering medication	Pitavastatin has shown potential anticancer properties against cervical cancer cells, triple-negative breast cancer cells, oral cancer cells, lung cancer cells, and angiogenesis. It targets molecular pathways involved in lung cancer pathogenesis, potentially promoting clinical use in the future.	[71, 93]
16.	Propranolol	Treat high blood pressure	Propranolol and betaxolol are active adrenoblockers against lung cancer cell lines A549 and H1299, inhibiting colony formation at 90% of EC50 value.	[69]
17.	Niclosamide	Anthelmintics	Niclosamide, a potent inhibitor of the AMPK/AKT/mTOR pathway, effectively suppresses tumor growth and induces autophagy in human lung cancer cells, making it a potential anti-NSCLC therapy candidate.	[94]
18.	Sertraline	Antidepressant	Sertraline, a cancer-sensitizing agent, has been shown to reduce tumor growth in lung cancer cell lines and interact with erlotinib, demonstrating anticancer activity through apoptosis, autophagy, and stem cell downregulation.	[95]
19.	Simvastatin	Treat high blood pressure	Simvastatin, an anticancer agent, inhibits proliferation and migration in non-small cell lung cancer, promotes apoptosis, and upregulates BIM expression, potentially improving lung cancer patient survival.	[95]
20.	Telmisartan	Treat high blood pressure, heart failure, and diabetic kidney disease.	Telmisartan, a new drug for treating NSCLC, inhibits PI3K/AKT signaling, preventing cell migration, and increases death receptor 5 expression, making TRAIL more effective in lung cancer treatment.	[96, 97]

Table 1.
List of drugs which are repurposed for LC.

S. No	Name	Description	Link	Ref
1.	BalestraWeb	BalestraWeb is a tool that uses latent factor models to predict drug-target interactions. The tool generates predictions with high confidence levels, with some interactions having a predicted score above 90%.	http://balestra.csb.pitt.edu/	[98]
2.	canSAR	It is a knowledge-base that integrates multidisciplinary data and machine learning for cancer drug discovery.	http://cansar.icr.ac.uk	[99]
3.	STITCH	Dispersed throughout the literature and various databases are details on biological pathways, drug-target relationships, and binding affinities.	http://stitch.embl.de/	[100]
4.	repoDB	A database containing details about medicines that have been approved and those that have not, along with their recommended uses.	http://apps.chiragjpgroup.org/repoDB/	[101]
5.	DT-Web	Using accessible clinical transcriptome datasets, DRUGSURV calculates medication effectiveness in patients with particular cancer subtypes.	https://alpha.dmi.unict.it/dtweb/	[102]

Table 2.
List of web-based tools for drug repositioning that are openly available.

8. Conclusions

This study utilized gene co-expression network analysis to identify potential drugs for NSCLC treatment. The bioinformatics task involves systematically identifying potential repositioning candidates using vast amounts of data generated by various techniques and domains. The study proposes crucial steps for an *in silico* drug repurposing pipeline to improve success rates. Drug repositioning is essential for improving pre-clinical drug development since it cuts costs and time when compared to conventional approaches. The development of computational drug repositioning methodologies has been expedited by the increasing availability of large-scale biological, biomedical, and electronic health-related data as well as high-performance computer capabilities. Finding novel therapeutic opportunities and cutting costs in comparison to conventional *de novo* drug development approaches depend on this procedure.

Conflict of interest

The authors declare no conflict of interest.

Author details

Sulekha Khute[1], Kareti Srinivasa Rao[2] and Paranthaman Subash[1*]

1 Department of Pharmacy, Sri Shanmugha College of Pharmacy, Salem, Tamil Nadu, India

2 Department of Pharmacy, Indira Gandhi National Tribal University, Amarkantak, Madhya Pradesh, India

*Address all correspondence to: subashpharm@gmail.com; subash.pharmacy@shanmugha.edu.in

References

[1] Borghaei H, Yim YM, Guerin A, Pivneva I, Shi S, Gandhi M, et al. Severe adverse events impact overall survival and costs in elderly patients with advanced non-small cell lung cancer on second-line therapy. Lung Cancer. 2018;**119**:112-119

[2] Youlden DR, Cramb SM, Baade PD. The international epidemiology of lung cancer: Geographical distribution and secular trends. Journal of Thoracic Oncology. 2008;**3**:819-831

[3] Lemjabbar-Alaoui H, Hassan OU, Yang Y-W, Buchanan P. Lung cancer: Biology and treatment options. Biochimica et Biophysica Acta. 2015;**1856**:189-210

[4] Wu L, Leng D, Cun D, Foged C, Yang M. Advances in combination therapy of lung cancer: Rationales, delivery technologies and dosage regimens. Journal of Controlled Release. 2017;**260**:78-91

[5] Ruiz-Ceja KA, Chirino YI. Current FDA-approved treatments for non-small cell lung cancer and potential biomarkers for its detection. Biomedicine and Pharmacotherapy. 2017;**90**:24-37

[6] Kim YH, Mishima M. Maintenance chemotherapy for non-small-cell lung cancer. Cancer Treatment Reviews. 2011;**37**:505-510

[7] Sandler A, Gray R, Perry MC, Brahmer J, Schiller JH, Dowlati A, et al. Paclitaxel–carboplatin alone or with bevacizumab for non-small-cell lung cancer. The New England Journal of Medicine. 2006;**355**:2542-2550

[8] Hanna N, Shepherd FA, Fossella FV, Pereira JR, De Marinis F, Von Pawel J, et al. Randomized phase III trial of pemetrexed versus docetaxel in patients with non–small-cell lung cancer previously treated with chemotherapy. Journal of Clinical Oncology. 2004;**22**:1589-1597

[9] Scagliotti GV, Parikh P, Von Pawel J, Biesma B, Vansteenkiste J, Manegold C, et al. Phase III study comparing cisplatin plus gemcitabine with cisplatin plus pemetrexed in chemotherapy-naive patients with advanced-stage non–small-cell lung cancer. Journal of Clinical Oncology. 2023;**41**:2458-2466

[10] Califano R, Romanidou O, Mountzios G, Landi L, Cappuzzo F, Blackhall F. Management of NSCLC disease progression after first-line EGFR tyrosine kinase inhibitors: What are the issues and potential therapies? Drugs. 2016;**76**:831-840

[11] Ciuleanu T, Stelmakh L, Cicenas S, Miliauskas S, Grigorescu AC, Hillenbach C, et al. Efficacy and safety of erlotinib versus chemotherapy in second-line treatment of patients with advanced, non-small-cell lung cancer with poor prognosis (TITAN): A randomised multicentre, open-label, phase 3 study. The Lancet Oncology Titan. 2012;**13**:300-308

[12] Pantziarka P, Bouche G, Meheus L, Sukhatme V, Sukhatme VP. Repurposing drugs in your medicine cabinet: Untapped opportunities for cancer therapy? Future Oncology. 2015;**11**:181-184

[13] Fojo T, Parkinson DR. Biologically targeted cancer therapy and marginal benefits: Are we making too much of too little or are we achieving too little by giving too much? Clinical Cancer Research. 2010;**16**:5972-5980

[14] Hay M, Thomas DW, Craighead JL, Economides C, Rosenthal J. Clinical development success rates for investigational drugs. Nature Biotechnology. 2014;**32**:40-51

[15] Paul SM, Mytelka DS, Dunwiddie CT, Persinger CC, Munos BH, Lindborg SR, et al. How to improve R&D productivity: The pharmaceutical industry's grand challenge. Nature Reviews. Drug Discovery. 2010;**9**:203-214

[16] Ashburn TT, Thor KB. Drug repositioning: Identifying and developing new uses for existing drugs. Nature Reviews. Drug Discovery. 2004;**3**:673-683

[17] Pushpakom S, Iorio F, Eyers PA, Jane Escott K, Hopper S, Wells A, et al. Drug repurposing: Progress, challenges and recommendations. Nature Reviews. Drug Discovery. 2019;**18**:41-58

[18] Ledford H. Coronavirus breakthrough: Dexamethasone is first drug shown to save lives. Nature. 2020;**582**:469

[19] Serafin MB, Bottega A, Foletto VS, da Rosa TF, Hörner A, Hörner R. Drug repositioning is an alternative for the treatment of coronavirus COVID-19. International Journal of Antimicrobial Agents. 2020;**55**:105969

[20] Harris M, Bhatti Y, Buckley J, Sharma D. Fast and frugal innovations in response to the COVID-19 pandemic. Nature Medicine. 2020;**26**:814-817

[21] Guy RK, DiPaola RS, Romanelli F, Dutch RE. Rapid repurposing of drugs for COVID-19. Science. 2020;**368**:829-830

[22] Iorio F, Bosotti R, Scacheri E, Belcastro V, Mithbaokar P, Ferriero R, et al. Discovery of drug mode of action and drug repositioning from transcriptional responses. Proceedings of the National Academy of Sciences of the United States of America. 2010;**107**:14621-14626

[23] Gloeckner C, Garner AL, Mersha F, Oksov Y, Tricoche N, Eubanks LM, et al. Repositioning of an existing drug for the neglected tropical disease onchocerciasis. Proceedings of the National Academy of Sciences of the United States of America. 2010;**107**:3424-3429

[24] Keiser MJ, Setola V, Irwin JJ, Laggner C, Abbas AI, Hufeisen SJ, et al. Predicting new molecular targets for known drugs. Nature. 2009;**462**:175-181

[25] Dudley JT, Deshpande T, Butte AJ. Exploiting drug–disease relationships for computational drug repositioning. Briefings in Bioinformatics. 2011;**12**:303-311

[26] Li J, Zheng S, Chen B, Butte AJ, Joshua Swamidass S, Zhiyong L. A survey of current trends in computational drug repositioning. Briefings in Bioinformatics. 2016;**17**:2-12

[27] Wu Z, Wang Y, Chen L. Network-based drug repositioning. Molecular BioSystems. 2013;**9**(6):1268-1281

[28] Jarada TN, Rokne JG, Alhajj R. A review of computational drug repositioning: Strategies, approaches, opportunities, challenges, and directions. Journal of Cheminformatics. 2020;**12**:1-23

[29] Keiser MJ, Setola V, Irwin JJ, Laggner C, Abbas AI, Hufeisen SJ, et al. Predicting new molecular targets for known drugs. Nature. 2009;**462**(7270):175-181

[30] Yamanishi Y, Araki M, Gutteridge A, Honda W, Kanehisa M. Prediction of drug–target interaction

networks from the integration of chemical and genomic spaces. Bioinformatics. 2008;**24**:i232-i240

[31] Zheng C, Guo Z, Huang C, Ziyin W, Li Y, Chen X, et al. Large-scale direct targeting for drug repositioning and discovery. Scientific Reports. 2015;**5**:11970

[32] Potti A, Mukherjee S, Petersen R, Dressman HK, Bild A, Koontz J, et al. A genomic strategy to refine prognosis in early-stage non–small-cell lung cancer. The New England Journal of Medicine. 2006;**355**:570-580

[33] Hu G, Agarwal P. Human disease-drug network based on genomic expression profiles. PLoS One. 2009;**4**:e6536

[34] Sirota M, Dudley JT, Kim J, Chiang AP, Morgan AA, Sweet-Cordero A, et al. Discovery and preclinical validation of drug indications using compendia of public gene expression data. Science Translational Medicine. 2011;**3**:96ra77

[35] Campillos M, Kuhn M, Gavin AC, Jensen LJ, Bork P. Drug target identification using side-effect similarity. Science. 2008;**321**(5886):263-266

[36] Sridhar D, Fakhraei S, Getoor L. A probabilistic approach for collective similarity-based drug–drug interaction prediction. Bioinformatics. 2016;**32**:3175-3182

[37] Yang L, Agarwal P. Systematic drug repositioning based on clinical side-effects. PLoS One. 2011;**6**:e28025

[38] Ye H, Liu Q, Wei J. Construction of drug network based on side effects and its application for drug repositioning. PLoS One. 2014;**9**(2):e87864

[39] Bisgin H, Liu Z, Fang H, Kelly R, Xiaowei X, Tong W. A phenome-guided drug repositioning through a latent variable model. BMC Bioinformatics. 2014;**15**:267

[40] Nugent T, Plachouras V, Leidner JL. Computational drug repositioning based on side-effects mined from social media. PeerJ Computer Science. 2016;**2**:e46

[41] Hoehndorf R, Oellrich A, Rebholz-Schuhmann D, Schofield PN, Gkoutos GV. Linking pharmGKB to phenotype studies and animal models of disease for drug repurposing. Pacific Symposium on Biocomputing. 2012:388-399

[42] Gottlieb A, Stein GY, Oron Y, Ruppin E, Sharan R. INDI: A computational framework for inferring drug interactions and their associated recommendations. Molecular Systems Biology. 2012;**8**:592

[43] Lim H, Poleksic A, Yao Y, Tong H, He D, Zhuang L, et al. Large-scale off-target identification using fast and accurate dual regularized one-class collaborative filtering and its application to drug repurposing. PLoS Computational Biology. 2016;**12**(10):e1005135

[44] Rakshit H, Chatterjee P, Roy D. A bidirectional drug repositioning approach for Parkinson's disease through network-based inference. Biochemical and Biophysical Research Communications. 2015;**457**(3):280-287

[45] Ozsoy MG, Özyer T, Polat F, Alhajj R. Realizing drug repositioning by adapting a recommendation system to handle the process. BMC Bioinformatics. 2018;**19**:1-14

[46] Yang CC, Zhao M. Mining heterogeneous network for drug

repositioning using phenotypic information extracted from social media and pharmaceutical databases. Artificial Intelligence in Medicine. 2019;**96**:80-92

[47] Zeng X, Zhu S, Liu X, Zhou Y, Nussinov R, Cheng F. DeepDR: A network-based deep learning approach to in silico drug repositioning. Bioinformatics. 2019;**35**(24):5191-5198

[48] Shim JS, Liu JO. Recent advances in drug repositioning for the discovery of new anticancer drugs. International Journal of Biological Sciences. 2014;**10**(7):654

[49] Sanseau P, Agarwal P, Barnes MR, Pastinen T, Richards JB, Cardon LR, et al. Use of genome-wide association studies for drug repositioning. Nature Biotechnology. 2012;**30**(4):317-320

[50] Greene CS, Voight BF. Pathway and network-based strategies to translate genetic discoveries into effective therapies. Human Molecular Genetics. 2016;**25**(R2):R94-R98

[51] Lu J, Chen L, Yin J, Huang T, Bi Y, Kong X, et al. Identification of new candidate drugs for lung cancer using chemical–chemical interactions, chemical–protein interactions and a K-means clustering algorithm. Journal of Biomolecular Structure and Dynamics. 2016;**34**(4):906-917

[52] Šubelj L, Bajec M. Unfolding communities in large complex networks: Combining defensive and offensive label propagation for core extraction. Physical Review E—Statistical, Nonlinear, and Soft Matter Physics. 2011;**83**(3):036103

[53] Yu L, Huang J, Ma Z, Zhang J, Zou Y, Gao L. Inferring drug-disease associations based on known protein complexes. BMC Medical Genomics. 2015;**8**:1-13

[54] Martínez V, Navarro C, Cano C, Fajardo W, Blanco A. DrugNet: Network-based drug–disease prioritization by integrating heterogeneous data. Artificial Intelligence in Medicine. 2015;**63**(1):41-49

[55] Hieronymus H, Lamb J, Ross KN, Peng XP, Clement C, Rodina A, et al. Gene expression signature-based chemical genomic prediction identifies a novel class of HSP90 pathway modulators. Cancer Cell. 2006;**10**(4):321-330

[56] Dudley JT, Sirota M, Shenoy M, Pai RK, Roedder S, Chiang AP, et al. Computational repositioning of the anticonvulsant topiramate for inflammatory bowel disease. Science Translational Medicine. 2011;**3**(96):96ra76-96ra76

[57] Sirota M, Dudley JT, Kim J, Chiang AP, Morgan AA, Sweet-Cordero A, et al. Discovery and preclinical validation of drug indications using compendia of public gene expression data. Science Translational Medicine. 17 Aug 2011;**3**(96):96ra77

[58] Oprea TI, Tropsha A, Faulon JL, Rintoul MD. Systems chemical biology. Nature Chemical Biology. 2007;**3**(8):447-450

[59] Dakshanamurthy S, Issa NT, Assefnia S, Seshasayee A, Peters OJ, Madhavan S, et al. Predicting new indications for approved drugs using a proteochemometric method. Journal of Medicinal Chemistry. 2012;**55**(15):6832-6848

[60] Teibo JO, Irozuru CE, Teibo TKA, Omotoso OE, Babalghith AO, Batiha GES. Perspective chapter: Appraisal of paclitaxel (taxol) pros and cons in the management of cancer–prospects in drug repurposing. In: Drug

Repurposing-Advances, Scopes and Opportunities in Drug Discovery. United Kingdom: IntechOpen; 2023

[61] Li J, Zhu X, Chen JY. Building disease-specific drug-protein connectivity maps from molecular interaction networks and PubMed abstracts. PLoS Computational Biology. 2009;**5**(7):e1000450

[62] Kaitin KI, DiMasi JA. Pharmaceutical innovation in the 21st century: New drug approvals in the first decade, 2000-2009. Clinical Pharmacology and Therapeutics. 2011;**89**(2):183-188

[63] Li YY, Jones SJ. Drug repositioning for personalized medicine. Genome Medicine. 2012;**4**:1-14

[64] Plodkowski RA, Nguyen Q, Sundaram U, Nguyen L, Chau DL, St. Jeor S. Bupropion and naltrexone: A review of their use individually and in combination for the treatment of obesity. Expert Opinion on Pharmacotherapy. 2009;**10**(6):1069-1081

[65] Caveney E, Caveney BJ, Somaratne R, Turner JR, Gourgiotis L. Pharmaceutical interventions for obesity: A public health perspective. Diabetes, Obesity and Metabolism. 2011;**13**(6):490-497

[66] Sam E, Athri P. Web-based drug repurposing tools: A survey. Briefings in Bioinformatics. 2019;**20**(1):299-316

[67] Min JS, Kwon S, Jin YH. SARS-CoV-2 RdRp inhibitors selected from a cell-based SARS-CoV-2 RdRp activity assay system. Biomedicine. 2021;**9**(8):996

[68] Zhou F, Du J, Wang J. Albendazole inhibits HIF-1α-dependent glycolysis and VEGF expression in non-small cell lung cancer cells. Molecular and Cellular Biochemistry. 2017;**428**:171-178

[69] Sidorova M, Petrikaitė V. The effect of beta adrenoreceptor blockers on viability and cell colony formation of non-small cell lung cancer cell lines A549 and H1299. Molecules. 2022;**27**(6):1938

[70] Amin F, Fathi F, Reiner Ž, Banach M, Sahebkar A. The role of statins in lung cancer. Archives of Medical Science: AMS. 2022;**18**(1):141

[71] Marcianò G, Palleria C, Casarella A, Rania V, Basile E, Catarisano L, et al. Effect of statins on lung cancer molecular pathways: A possible therapeutic role. Pharmaceuticals. 2022;**15**(5):589

[72] Xie F, Gong J, Tan H, Zhang H, Ma J. Preclinical evidence of synergism between atovaquone and chemotherapy by AMPK-dependent mitochondrial dysfunction. European Journal of Pharmacology. 2021;**907**:174256

[73] Chen L, He Y, Huang H, Liao H, Wei W. Selective COX-2 inhibitor celecoxib combined with EGFR-TKI ZD1839 on non-small cell lung cancer cell lines: In vitro toxicity and mechanism study. Medical Oncology. 2008;**25**:161-171

[74] Liu X, Yue P, Zhou Z, Khuri FR, Sun SY. Death receptor regulation and celecoxib-induced apoptosis in human lung cancer cells. Journal of the National Cancer Institute. 2004;**96**(23):1769-1780

[75] De Groot DJA, De Vries EGE, Groen HJM, De Jong S. Non-steroidal anti-inflammatory drugs to potentiate chemotherapy effects: From lab to clinic. Critical Reviews in Oncology/Hematology. 2007;**61**(1):52-69

[76] Kato T, Fujino H, Oyama S, Kawashima T, Murayama T. Indomethacin induces cellular morphological change and migration via epithelial-mesenchymal transition in A549

human lung cancer cells: A novel cyclooxygenase-inhibition-independent effect. Biochemical Pharmacology. 2011;**82**(11):1781-1791

[77] López-Contreras F, Muñoz-Uribe M, Pérez-Laines J, Ascencio-Leal L, Rivera-Dictter A, Martin-Martin A, et al. Searching for drug synergy against cancer through polyamine metabolism impairment: Insight into the metabolic effect of indomethacin on lung cancer cells. Frontiers in Pharmacology. 2020;**10**:1670

[78] Parvathaneni V, Shukla SK, Gupta V. Development and characterization of folic acid-conjugated amodiaquine-loaded nanoparticles–efficacy in cancer treatment. Pharmaceutics. 2023;**15**(3):1001

[79] Aftab BT, Dobromilskaya I, Liu JO, Rudin CM. Itraconazole inhibits angiogenesis and tumor growth in non–small cell lung cancer. Cancer Research. 2011;**71**(21):6764-6772

[80] Mohamed AW, Elbassiouny M, Elkhodary DA, Shawki MA, Saad AS. The effect of itraconazole on the clinical outcomes of patients with advanced non-small cell lung cancer receiving platinum-based chemotherapy: A randomized controlled study. Medical Oncology. 2021;**38**:1-9

[81] Li CL, Fang ZX, Wu Z, Hou YY, Wu HT, Liu J. Repurposed itraconazole for use in the treatment of malignancies as a promising therapeutic strategy. Biomedicine and Pharmacotherapy. 2022;**154**:113616

[82] Qiao X, Wang C, Wang W, Shang Y, Li Y, Ni J, et al. Levamisole enhances DR4-independent apoptosis induced by TRAIL through inhibiting the activation of JNK in lung cancer. Life Sciences. 2020;**257**:118034

[83] Stevenson HC, Green I, Hamilton JM, Calabro BA, Parkinson DR. Levamisole: Known effects on the immune system, clinical results, and future applications to the treatment of cancer. Journal of Clinical Oncology. 1991;**9**(11):2052-2066

[84] Marima R, Hull R, Dlamini Z, Penny C. Efavirenz and lopinavir/ritonavir alter cell cycle regulation in lung cancer. Frontiers in Oncology. 2020;**10**:1693

[85] Sanli T, Liu C, Rashid A, Hopmans SN, Tsiani E, Schultz C, et al. Lovastatin sensitizes lung cancer cells to ionizing radiation: Modulation of molecular pathways of radioresistance and tumor suppression. Journal of Thoracic Oncology. 2011;**6**(3):439-450

[86] Fatehi Hassanabad A, MacQueen KT. Molecular mechanisms underlining the role of metformin as a therapeutic agent in lung cancer. Cellular Oncology. 2021;**44**:1-18

[87] Li C, Xue Y, Xi YR, Xie K. Progress in the application and mechanism of metformin in treating non-small cell lung cancer. Oncology Letters. 2017;**13**(5):2873-2880

[88] Liang Z, Chen Q, Pan L, She X, Chen T. Mebendazole induces apoptosis and inhibits migration via the reactive oxygen species-mediated STAT3 signaling downregulation in non-small cell lung cancer. Journal of Thoracic Disease. 2024;**16**(2):1412

[89] Elayapillai S, Ramraj S, Benbrook DM, Bieniasz M, Wang L, Pathuri G, et al. Potential and mechanism of mebendazole for treatment and maintenance of ovarian cancer. Gynecologic Oncology. 2021;**160**(1):302-311

[90] Yang L, Yang J, Liu H, Lan J, Xu Y, Wu X, et al. Minocycline binds and

inhibits LYN activity to prevent STAT3-meditated metastasis of colorectal cancer. International Journal of Biological Sciences. 2022;**18**(6):2540

[91] Ko JC, Wang TJ, Chang PY, Syu JJ, Chen JC, Chen CY, et al. Minocycline enhances mitomycin C-induced cytotoxicity through down-regulating ERK1/2-mediated Rad51 expression in human non-small cell lung cancer cells. Biochemical Pharmacology. 2015;**97**(3):331-340

[92] Ciaramella V, Sasso FC, Di Liello R, Corte CMD, Barra G, Viscardi G, et al. Activity and molecular targets of pioglitazone via blockade of proliferation, invasiveness and bioenergetics in human NSCLC. Journal of Experimental and Clinical Cancer Research. 2019;**38**:1-13

[93] Chen YH, Wu JX, Yang SF, Wu YC, Hsiao YH. Molecular mechanisms underlying the anticancer properties of pitavastatin against cervical cancer cells. International Journal of Molecular Sciences. 2024;**25**(14):7915

[94] Chai WH, Li YR, Lin SH, Chao YH, Chen CH, Chan PC, et al. Antihelminthic niclosamide induces autophagy and delayed apoptosis in human non-small lung cancer cells in vitro and in vivo. Anticancer Research. 2020;**40**(3):1405-1417

[95] Duarte D, Vale N. Antidepressant drug sertraline against human cancer cells. Biomolecules. 2022;**12**(10):1513

[96] Rasheduzzaman M, Moon JH, Lee JH, Nazim UM, Park SY. Telmisartan generates ROS-dependent upregulation of death receptor 5 to sensitize TRAIL in lung cancer via inhibition of autophagy flux. The International Journal of Biochemistry and Cell Biology. 2018;**102**:20-30

[97] Zhang S, Wang Y. Telmisartan inhibits NSCLC A549 cell proliferation and migration by regulating the PI3K/AKT signaling pathway. Oncology Letters. 2018;**15**(4):5859-5864

[98] Cobanoglu MC, Oltvai ZN, Taylor DL, Bahar I. BalestraWeb: Efficient online evaluation of drug–target interactions. Bioinformatics. 2015;**31**(1):131-133

[99] Bulusu KC, Tym JE, Coker EA, Schierz AC, Al-Lazikani B. canSAR: Updated cancer research and drug discovery knowledgebase. Nucleic Acids Research. 2014;**42**(D1):D1040-D1047

[100] Szklarczyk D, Santos A, Von Mering C, Jensen LJ, Bork P, Kuhn M. STITCH 5: Augmenting protein–chemical interaction networks with tissue and affinity data. Nucleic Acids Research. 2016;**44**(D1):D380-D384

[101] Brown AS, Patel CJ. A standard database for drug repositioning. Scientific Data. 2017;**4**(1):1-7

[102] Alaimo S, Bonnici V, Cancemi D, Ferro A, Giugno R, Pulvirenti A. DT-web: A web-based application for drug-target interaction and drug combination prediction through domain-tuned network-based inference. BMC Systems Biology. 2015;**9**:1-11

Chapter 6

Repurposing Niclosamide for Treatment of Acute Myeloid Leukemia and Other Diseases

Namrata Patel, Kailen Mark, Adam Frymoyer, Norman Lacayo and Kathleen M. Sakamoto

Abstract

Niclosamide (NIC) is a salicylanilide that was developed for treatment of tapeworms and other parasitic infections. The mechanism of action is primarily to inhibit oxidative phosphorylation. However, more recently, additional signaling pathways and targets have been identified. Pre-clinical studies have demonstrated that NIC has potential effects in treating infectious diseases, diabetic kidney disease, cardiovascular diseases, and cancer. This chapter summarizes the pharmacology and recent pre-clinical and clinical studies of NIC. Further studies are needed to determine whether NIC can be repurposed to treat acute myeloid leukemia, prostate cancer, SARS-CoV-2, hepatitis E virus, diabetic kidney disease, hepatitis virus, rheumatoid arthritis, and heart failure.

Keywords: Niclosamide, tapeworms, oxidative phosphorylation, pre-clinical studies, cancer, acute myeloid leukemia

1. Introduction

NIC (5-chloro-N-(2-chloro-4-nitrophenyl)-2-hydroxybenzamide) is a salicylanilide marketed under the brand name Yomesan® from Europe as an oral anthelmintic drug to treat parasitic infections. It was originally discovered at Bayer in 1953 and later developed as a molluscicide to kill snails, an intermediate host of schistosomiasis. Mechanistically, NIC uncouples oxidative phosphorylation in the cell mitochondria, perturbing the production of adenosine triphosphate, resulting in impaired parasitic motility [1–3]. NIC was approved by the US FDA for use in humans to treat tapeworm infections in 1982. Albeit voluntarily withdrawn by Bayer from the US market in 1996 due to limited profitability, it is currently included within the World Health Organization's list of essential medicines and marketed as an anti-helminthic in many other countries [4]. Even though its widespread use has been limited due to low aqueous solubility and poor systemic bioavailability, pre-clinical studies have evidenced multiple cellular targets of NIC, making it a desirable agent for drug repurposing [3]. Consequently, it is being investigated for indications ranging from viral and bacterial infections and inflammatory airway diseases to metabolic diseases and cancers. Additionally, in order to capitalize on the vast pharmacological potential of NIC, several new formulations are being trialed at the pre-clinical and clinical stages with an aim to overcome its low solubility and bioavailability. This chapter aims to highlight the ongoing efforts to repurpose NIC for a multitude of indications using the parent and newer formulations.

2. Clinical pharmacology

NIC is a derivative of salicylic acid, a salicylanilide belonging to a large group of lipophilic, weakly acidic molecules (**Figure 1**) [5].

A significant portion of NIC's therapeutic efficacy is derived from its inhibition of oxidative phosphorylation. It is a weakly acidic lipophilic protonophore that translocates protons across the mitochondrial membrane, resulting in mitochondrial uncoupling and futile cycles of glucose and fatty acid oxidation. Its action as a mild mitochondrial uncoupler is sufficient to kill tapeworms residing in the gastrointestinal tract. It has demonstrated an excellent safety profile in humans as transient mild mitochondrial uncoupling is tolerable in normal cells [6]. In addition to this classic mode of action, recent scientific literature has illuminated a myriad of pathways through which NIC can exert its effects. Pre-clinical studies have reported NIC-driven modulation of Wingless-related integration site (Wnt)/(beta-catenin) β-catenin, mammalian target of rapamycin complex 1 (mTORC1), Signal transducer and activator of transcription 3 (STAT3), Nuclear factor kappa B (NF-κB), cyclic AMP Response Element Binding Protein (CREB), and Neurogenic locus notch homolog protein 1 (Notch 1) signaling pathways [3].

The lipophilic characteristic of the drug restricts its aqueous solubility and systemic bioavailability. The solubility of NIC has been reported in the range of 0.2–19 mg/L, whereas the solubility of its ethanolamine salt (NEN) ranges from 145 to 372 mg/L [7]. Oral NIC, marketed as a chewable tablet, is only partially absorbed from the intestinal tract with a bioavailability of 5.5–10%. It is rapidly eliminated by the kidneys with no cumulative toxic effects [5]. The plasma half-life of NIC is short at about 6 hours [8], and therefore when systemic exposure is needed, twice daily or thrice daily administration will be indicated. Distribution studies in rodents with oral doses of 40 mg/kg NIC ethanolamine, (i.e., ~34 mg/kg NIC) and 50 mg/kg NIC demonstrate that tissue levels are highest in excretory organs (intestines, liver, and kidney) and low to negligible levels are achieved in other tissues (such as the brain, heart, and lungs) [5]. The adult dose of NIC as an anthelmintic is 2 grams (g). The serum concentration of NIC after a single oral dose of 2 g leads to maximal serum concentrations of 0.25–6.0 mcg/mL [7]. NIC is a safe drug when orally administered, but injection (intraperitoneally and intravenously) of the drug can lead to adverse effects (hypopnea, sedation, and convulsions) [8].

To date, a limited number of studies have analyzed the metabolic profile of NIC. Some published reports have noted a possible involvement of uridine

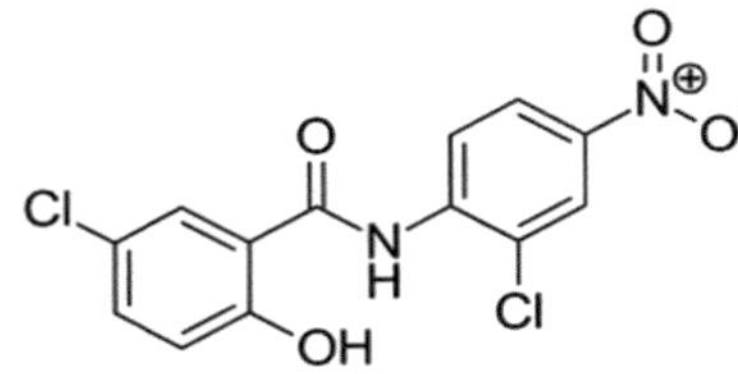

Figure 1.
NIC (5-chloro-N-(2-chloro-4-nitrophenyl)-2-hydroxybenzamide).

5′-diphospho-glucuronosyltransferase1A1 (UGT1A1), a Phase II polymorphic enzyme, in the metabolism and/or bio-transformation of this agent. One of these studies also associated NIC disposition with cytochrome P450 1A2-mediated hydroxylation [8]. The effect of NIC on Phase I or Phase II enzymes (i.e., induction or inhibition) has not yet been completely elucidated and is actively being investigated. A study by Hamdoun, et al., observed that NIC inhibited glutathione synthetase (GS) [9]. Consequently, this could attenuate the production of glutathione (GSH), a cofactor required for Phase II metabolism of drugs such as busulfan, cisplatin, and acetaminophen. Interestingly, GSH is also known to be involved in the development of drug resistance via its antioxidant property of scavenging reactive oxygen species (ROS). Through its inhibition of GSH, NIC could exhibit a therapeutic role in multidrug-resistant cancers, including leukemia.

3. Potential applications of NIC: pre-clinical data

Several studies have examined the role of NIC as a potential therapeutic option for microbial infections. The COVID-19 pandemic provided an impetus to unlock its antiviral potential against the SARS-CoV-2 virus based on data from cellular experiments and its relatively favorable adverse effect profile. NIC is presumed to mediate its therapeutic activity in this setting through inhibition of TransMEMbraine Protein 16 (TMEM16), a calcium-activated chloride channel protein found to mediate viral spike-induced syncytia formation in SARS-CoV-2 infections, induction of autophagy, and its protonophoric activity. The latter two have been purported to play a role in preventing viral replication by interfering with viral entry and egress via endosomal neutralization [5, 10]. A pre-clinical study by Vazquez-Rodriguez et al. highlighted the antibacterial efficacy of NIC against biofilm-associated microbes, *Staphylococcus aureus* and *Staphylococcus epidermidis* in catheter-related bloodstream infections (CRBSIs) [11]. A time-kill study by Rajamuthiah demonstrated that NIC is bacteriostatic [12]. NIC encapsulated in a nanoparticle was shown to prevent *Candida albicans (C. albicans)* hyphenation and early biofilm growth and disengaged fully grown biofilms of drug-resistant *C. albicans* and *Candida auris* from their growth surface, thus highlighting its role as a potential antifungal agent as well. Here, NIC was postulated to inhibit Ndu1, a *C. albicans* protein essential for mitochondrial respiration [13].

Inflammatory airway diseases, such as asthma, cystic fibrosis (CF), and chronic obstructive pulmonary disease (COPD), are characterized by mucus hypersecretion and airway plugging. The TMEM16A protein has been detected in mucus-producing club/goblet cells and airway smooth muscle as well where it contributes to mucus hypersecretion and bronchoconstriction. This has paved the way for examining NIC as a potential treatment of inflammatory airway disease [14].

NIC may also play a therapeutic role in the treatment of chronic inflammatory autoimmune diseases such as rheumatoid arthritis (RA), given its observed anti-inflammatory effect in pre-clinical studies. In their in-vitro and mouse model study, Liang and colleagues observed that NIC attenuated the secretion of several interleukins including IL-1β, IL-6, IL-8, IL-7A, and interferon-γ (INF-γ) from tumor necrosis factor-α (TNF-α) stimulated RA fibroblast-like synoviocytes (FLS) in a dose-dependent manner. NIC also inhibited TNF-α-induced extracellular signal-regulated kinase (ERK) and c-Jun N-terminal kinase (JNK) phosphorylation, kinases reported to have an important role in chronic synovitis in RA. The group reported a reduction in the severity of collagen-induced arthritis (CIA) in their NIC-treated mouse model as well.

Based on their findings, they further postulated that the mechanism of the inhibitory effect of NIC on TNF-α-induced interleukins might be mediated by nuclear factor kappa B (NF-κB) signaling pathway [15]. Another group evaluated the anti-rheumatoid activity of oral NIC in collagen-induced arthritic rats. In this study, diclofenac, a common RA non-steroidal anti-inflammatory drug, served as a comparator group to two different dose levels of NIC (50 mg/kg and 100 mg/kg). A significant reduction in inflammatory markers of TNF-α and IL-1β and the resultant decline in arthritic symptoms was noted in the higher dose NIC group. These observations were generally comparable to the diclofenac group [16].

The therapeutic potential of NIC is also being explored in the realm of metabolic disorders. Preliminary studies have indicated that NIC ethanolamine salt (NEN) could help with regulating insulin resistance in Type II Diabetes via increased lipid oxidation through mitochondrial uncoupling [17]. It was recently discovered that multiple genes of the renin-angiotensin-aldosterone system (RAAS) are direct downstream targets of the Wnt/β-catenin pathway. NIC has been reported to be a potent inhibitor of Wnt/β-catenin. Additionally, pre-clinical studies showed that NIC could improve diabetes and diabetic kidney disease (DKD) through inhibition of the mammalian target of rapamycin (mTOR) signaling pathway that is implicated in diabetes and DKD progression [18].

NIC has also been reported to potentially prevent or slow the progression of renal fibrosis. The phosphate form of NIC reduced proteinuria, glomerulosclerotic lesions, and interstitial fibrosis in a murine model of adriamycin nephrology, primarily through inhibition of Transforming Growth Factor (TGF)-beta-induced expression of homeodomain-interacting protein kinase 2 [19]. Renal ischemia and reperfusion injury could be protected by NIC by altering the expression levels of autophagy-associated proteins in rat kidneys [20]. End-stage renal disease caused by inflammation and fibrosis mediated by STAT3 and protein tyrosine phosphatase-1B could also be potentially decreased with NIC [21]. Therefore, NIC is a potential drug for a variety of renal diseases.

Another virus that has been identified to be responsive to NIC is hepatitis. The Hepatitis E virus causes acute hepatitis in immunocompromised individuals. NIC inhibits hepatitis E through inhibition of NFκB signaling pathways. This inhibition is independent of STAT3 [22]. Thus, NIC could potentially be repurposed to treat hepatitis infections. Future clinical trials are necessary to demonstrate the efficacy of NIC in patients with Hepatitis E and other viral infections [23].

Because of its effects on mitochondrial activity, NIC has been proposed as a potential treatment for heart failure. Pre-clinical studies have demonstrated that NIC increases mitochondrial respiration and adenosine triphosphate production in cardiomyocytes and improves heart failure in mice by decreasing inflammation [24]. NIC has also been demonstrated to decrease artery constriction [25]. Another study reported that NIC treatment augmented the endothelium-dependent relaxation of the thoracic aorta in diabetic rats [26]. Therefore, there are several potential trials to study the effects of NIC in cardiovascular disease.

In numerous pre-clinical studies, NIC has been shown to attenuate malignant cell growth by targeting a variety of oncogenic pathways. As a result, it has been identified as a potential anticancer agent that exerts cytotoxic and cytostatic activity against a wide range of cancer types including leukemia, breast cancer, prostate cancer, colorectal cancer, hepatocellular carcinoma, renal cell carcinoma, and glioblastoma. In colorectal cancer cells, NIC was observed to decrease the expression of disheveled segment polarity protein-2 (Dvl-2) and proto-oncogene β-catenin, as well as to prevent the association between β-catenin and T-cell factor (TCF) [27–31]. In prostate cancer, NIC has been found to target androgen receptor (AR) variant 7 (AR-V7) and inhibit STAT3 phosphorylation via IL-6 to attenuate prostate cancer growth [32]. Targeting of NOTCH, mTOR, and NF-κB signaling cascades by NIC in other cancer groups has also demonstrated pre-clinical response with some evidence that it may improve immunotherapy by modulating pathways such as Programmed Cell Death Protein (PD-1)/Programmed Cell Death Ligand 1 (PDL-1) [5, 33]. In acute myelogenous leukemia (AML), NIC has been shown to induce caspase-dependent apoptosis by inhibiting the NF-kβ and increasing ROS levels [34]. In pediatric leukemia, NIC was found to inhibit CREB function and CREB-mediated gene expression in cells [35].

4. NIC and acute myeloid leukemia

Acute myeloid leukemia (AML) is a malignancy of the bone marrow characterized by the aberrant proliferation of immature myeloid cells. The accumulation of genomic and epigenetic abnormalities drives the dysregulation of self-renewal and uncontrolled growth. The overall 5-year survival rate is ~30%, but older patients have poorer outcomes with a much lower 5-year survival rate at less than 10% [36, 37]. Standard of care is induction therapy known as the "7 + 3 regimen" consisting of 7 days of cytarabine and 3 days of an anthracycline such as daunorubicin. However, this intensive therapy can lead to significant toxicities and morbidity.

The rapid growth of cancer cells requires massive amounts of metabolites and energy, and this demand is fulfilled by dysregulated metabolic signatures. One classic example is the Warburg effect, which occurs in many types of cancers including leukemia. A century ago, the German physician Otto Warburg discovered that cancer cells can upregulate glycolysis instead of oxidative phosphorylation to produce the energy required for rapid proliferation. Immature myeloid blasts are produced by a small, quiescent population of leukemic stem cells (LSCs), which are more resistant to standard induction chemotherapy than dividing blast cells [38]. While leukemic blasts utilize the Warburg effect and upregulate glycolysis to proliferate, LSCs rely on oxidative phosphorylation to maintain their quiescence. High oxidative phosphorylation contributes to chemotherapy resistance in LSCs and AML blasts [39]. Therefore, inhibition of oxidative phosphorylation has the potential to target LSCs and re-sensitize myeloid blasts to conventional chemotherapy. Thus, the targeting of dysregulated metabolic signatures in AML is a potential avenue for novel therapies.

The antineoplastic mechanism of NIC has not been fully elucidated in acute myeloid leukemia (AML) but some studies have found that the ability of NIC to uncouple oxidative phosphorylation in helminths can also occur in AML cells. In adrenocortical carcinoma cells, treatment with NIC decreases the oxygen consumption rate and extracellular acidification rate, which is indicative of electron transport chain uncoupling [40]. A reduction in mitochondrial membrane potential occurs within 3 hours of NIC treatment. In stem-like ovarian cancer cells, NIC downregulates genes involved in oxidative phosphorylation and increases the production of reactive oxygen species (ROS) [41]. NIC also induces fragmentation of mitochondria and leads to autophagy and apoptosis in HeLa cells [42]. NIC was also previously reported to inhibit Notch signaling and tumor necrosis factor-mediated NF-$_{K}$B-dependent gene transcription in AML [34]. AML cells treated with NIC have increased ROS production. These findings highlight NIC as a potential therapy for a wide range of malignancies through inhibition of several signaling pathways.

4.1 CREB as a target for AML

The cyclic AMP response element binding protein (CREB) is a leucine zipper transcription factor that regulates several cellular functions including metabolism, cell cycle, and cell survival in both hematopoietic and neuronal cells. CREB is overexpressed AML cells compared to healthy bone marrow stem cells and this was associated with a worse prognosis [43].

Overexpression of CREB is a driver of abnormal proliferation and survival in AML. AML cells have a 2- to 3-fold increase in CREB protein and messenger ribonucleic acid (mRNA) when compared to healthy and non-leukemic controls, and CREB overexpression is associated with a worse prognosis [44]. Myeloid leukemia cell lines transfected to overexpress CREB have an elevated growth rate and an increase in the number of cells in the S phase of the cell cycle. Transgenic mice with CREB overexpressed in the myeloid lineage develop myeloproliferative syndrome and have more robust self-renewal of the bone marrow progenitors in methylcellulose colony assays, independent of growth factors. Conversely, CREB knockdown significantly reduces the viability and inhibits the growth of AML cells. In mouse transduction/transplantation experiments, knockdown of CREB in healthy mouse hematopoietic stem and progenitor cells results in normal long-term engraftment with little effects on short-term engraftment [43]. Therefore, CREB overexpression contributes to the proliferative phenotype of AML blasts, and CREB is a potential therapeutic target for AML.

CREB is activated by phosphorylation on serine 133 by several kinases including PP90 ribosomal S6 kinase, mitogen-activated protein kinase kinase (MEKK), protein kinase A, and calmodulin kinases [45]. Upon phosphorylation, the kinase-inducible domain (KID) of CREB is conformationally folded to interact with the kinase-inducible acceptor domain (KIX) of the co-activator CREB binding protein (CBP). This CREB/CBP complex then binds to DNA at consensus sites known as the conserved cAMP-responsive elements (CREs) to mediate transcription of its target genes. There are several genes containing CRE motifs involved in cellular processes including metabolism, glucose homeostasis, cell proliferation, survival, cell cycle, and differentiation. The development of small molecules to inhibit CREB activity via KIX:KID interaction revealed NIC as a potent CREB inhibitor.

4.2 CREB inhibitors

(See **Figure 2**)

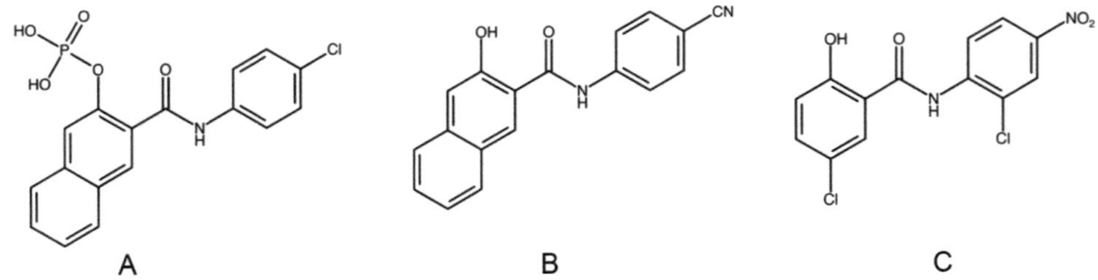

Figure 2.
CREB inhibitors. Three previously published structures of compounds that inhibit CREB are shown, including (A) KG501 [46], (B) XX-650-23 [47], and (C) NIC [35].

4.2.1 KG-501

An NMR-based library screen consisting of over 760 compounds for KIX binding identified the first potent CREB inhibitor, napthol-AS-E-phosphate (**Figure 2A**) [46]. KG-501 directly interacts with the KIX region of CBP at key residues in the KIX:KID interface between residues R600 and V608 with a K_i of ~90 μM. Transcription of endogenous CREB target genes such as nuclear receptor subfamily 4 group A member 2 (NR4A2), c-fos, and Regulator of G-protein signaling 2 (RGS2) is reduced at 10 μM of KG-501. KG-501 also inhibits CBP binding to other transcription factors with similar structures including NF-κB and Myb.

Further studies revealed that KG-501 is not stable in culture media and has low cell permeability. KG-501 served as a proof-of-concept that blocking the KIX:KID interaction can effectively disrupt CREB-mediated gene transcription. The structure provided a backbone for the development of more potent inhibitors with improved specificity to CREB.

4.2.2 XX-650-23

Investigation of the structure-activity relationship (SAR) between KG-501 and the KIX domain identified key components for binding and led to the development of small molecule XX-650-23 (**Figure 2B**) [47]. This molecule inhibits KIX:KID binding with a 50% inhibitory concentration (IC50) of 3.20 ± 0.43 μM, as measured by split Renilla luciferase complementation assay, and inhibits CREB-mediated transcription in a dose-dependent manner. RNA-seq analysis found no significant change in the target genes of other transcription factors that bind to CPB such as myeloblastosis viral oncogene homolog (Myb), v-rel avian reticuloendotheliosis viral oncogene homolog A (RelA), -rel avian reticuloendotheliosis viral oncogene homolog B (RelB), Forkhead box O3 (Foxo3), and Forkhead box O1 (Foxo1), indicating that XX-650-23 specifically inhibits CBP binding only to CREB. Treatment of AML cell lines and human AML patient samples with XX-650-23 potently reduces cell viability with no significant toxicity to normal human hematopoietic cells up to 10 μM. XX-650-23 induces apoptosis of AML cells through activation of the intrinsic apoptosis pathway and reduction of the CREB-regulated anti-apoptotic blocks programmed cell death (BCL2) family protein levels. Regulators of the cell cycle, such as cyclins and replication factor C2 (RFC2), are downregulated upon XX-650-23 treatment, causing AML cells to undergo cell cycle arrest at the G1/S cell cycle transition. In AML cell line and AML patient-derived xenograft mouse models, mice treated with XX-650-23 had a reduction in leukemia cell engraftment, reduced disease burden, and significantly greater median survival. However, due to physical properties such as low solubility and a short half-life in mice, XX-650-23 is not a suitable candidate for clinical applications. Additional compounds were developed to optimize XX-650-23 through SAR [48].

4.2.3 NIC as a CREB inhibitor in AML

A search for FDA-approved structural analog of XX-650-23 led to the identification of NIC (**Figure 2C**) as a candidate for CREB inhibition [35, 48]. NIC shares a similar chemical structure with XX-650-23 including a salicylamide core and electron-withdrawing groups para to the phenol hydroxyl group and anilide. Using a Renilla luciferase complementation assay, NIC was found to interact with the KIX:KID domain more potently than XX-650-23.

Treatment of AML cell lines and patient samples with NIC reduces cell viability in a dose-dependent manner with IC50 values of 0.28–0.51 μM [35]. NIC induces apoptosis in the LSC population and inhibits colony formation of AML blasts in methylcellulose culture with an IC50 of 19.8 nM [48]. NIC does not exhibit toxicity to colony formation of healthy bone marrow up to 10 μM, indicating a wide therapeutic window. Immunocompromised mice injected with AML cell lines [34] and AML patient samples [35] demonstrated that NIC decreases engraftment of leukemia cells and leukemic burden, and increases the median survival of mice compared to vehicle. Sequential treatment of AML cells with NIC and cytarabine or daunorubicin also results in a synergistic cytotoxic effect, indicating that pretreatment of NIC can potentially enhance sensitivity to conventional chemotherapy.

NIC inhibits CREB-mediated transcription in AML and induces apoptosis. CREB knockdown in AML cell lines protects cells from the cytotoxic effect of NIC and shifts the dose-response curve to the right, indicating that one potential mechanism of NIC is CREB inhibition. CREB-mediated transcription is decreased by NIC treatment with an IC50 of 1.24 μM in AML cell lines. Similar to XX-650-23, NIC induces cell cycle arrest at the G1 phase by reducing CREB-mediated transcription of replication factor C subunit 3 (RFC3) and DNA polymerase delta subunit (POLD2).

These pre-clinical findings have supported the development of a Phase 1 clinical trial to evaluate the effects of NIC in combination with cytarabine in AML patients.

5. Clinical trials

5.1 Cancer

The therapeutic potential of NIC and its novel formulations in cancer has been investigated/explored in early-phase clinical trials for adults with metastatic prostate and colorectal cancer. In addition, it is being explored in pediatrics for relapsed AML.

A recent Phase 1b clinical trial of NIC in combination with abiraterone and prednisone in men with castration-resistant prostate cancer (CRPC) reported the safety and clinical activity of NIC use in this patient population. The primary objective of the trial was to identify a maximum tolerated dose (MTD) and recommended phase 2 dose (RP2D) of a novel reformulated orally bioavailable, NIC (PDMX1001). All patients enrolled in the trial were treated with abiraterone acetate 1000 mg by mouth (PO) daily and prednisone 5 mg PO twice a day (bid), starting the same day when NIC was started for 28 days. The first dose level (DL 0) was dosed at 400 mg PO BID of NIC with targeted escalation to dose level 4 dose of 1600 mg PO TID. Overall, nine patients with metastatic CRPC (mCRPC) were accrued in the trial with treatment cycles ranging from 1 cycle to over 42 cycles (median 6 cycles). The recommended Phase II dose of NIC/PDMX1001 was 1200 mg orally three times daily (DL 3). Trough and peak NIC concentrations exceeded the therapeutic threshold of>0.2 microgram per microliter. The combination was found to be well tolerated with the most frequent adverse effect of diarrhea. Grade 3 toxicities observed included abdominal pain, fatigue, hypoalbuminemia, and anorexia. For Grade 1–2 events, diarrhea, fatigue, headache, and anorexia were the most common [49].

Another Phase 1 trial studied NIC in combination with enzalutamide in men with castration-resistant prostate cancer [50]. The primary objective was to assess safety. NIC was given three times daily (TID) at the following dose levels: 500, 1000, or 1500 mg. There were no dose-limiting toxicities (DLTs) in three patients on the 500 mg TID cohort; however, both (N = 2) subjects on the 1000 mg TID cohort experienced DLTs (prolonged grade 3 nausea, vomiting, diarrhea; and colitis). The maximum plasma concentration ranged from 35.7 to 182 ng/mL and was not consistently above the minimum effective concentration in pre-clinical studies. The study was closed as plasma concentrations at the maximum tolerated dose (500 mg TID) were not consistently above the expected therapeutic threshold.

The Phase II NIKOLO trial investigated the safety and efficacy of orally applied NIC in patients with metachronous or synchronous metastases of colorectal cancer progressing after therapy. The primary objective of the study was progression-free survival (PFS) after 4 months. All patients received 2 grams PO daily of NIC until progression or unacceptable toxicity. The study is ongoing, but no drug-related toxicities have been reported so far [28].

A Phase 1 trial of NIC in pediatric and young adult patients with relapsed or refractory AML is ongoing. The primary objective of the study is to identify and evaluate safety for the recommended phase 2 dose (RP2D) of NIC in combination with cytarabine for relapsed and/or refractory acute myeloid leukemia (AML). NIC will be administered orally twice daily for 14 days (Days 1 to 14) starting at Level 1 (500 mg/m^2/day divided PO BID) in a 28-day cycle. Depending upon observed dose limiting toxicities (DLT), the dose will get escalated up to dose level 3 (1200 mg/m^2/day divided BID). Each dose level will be followed by backbone chemotherapy: Cytarabine 2000 mg/m^2 IV daily over 4 hours on Days 15–19 [51].

5.2 Metabolic disorders

A randomized clinical trial explored the efficacy of NIC as an adjuvant therapy in diabetic kidney disease. The study subjects were randomized to either NIC plus Ramipril or just Ramipril for 6 months. The primary outcomes included changes in urinary albumin to creatinine ratio (UACR), serum creatinine, and estimated glomerular filtration rate (eGFR). The secondary outcomes were measurements of urinary matrix metalloproteinase-7 (MMP-7), 8-hydroxy-2′-deoxyguanosine (8-OHdG), and podocalyxin (PCX). Patients in the NIC arm received ramipril plus NIC 1 g once daily, and patients in the control arm received ramipril only for 6 months. Overall, 41 patients were recruited for each arm, with 30 patients completing the study on each arm of the trial. The addition of NIC to patients with diabetic kidney disease receiving an angiotensin-converting enzyme inhibitor significantly reduces albumin excretion. The NIC arm showed a 24.2% decrease in baseline albumin to creatinine excretion (95% CI, −30 to −18.3%), in contrast to the control arm, which showed an 11.1% increase in baseline UACR (95% CI, 4 to 18.2%). In addition, patients who received NIC preserved their serum creatinine and eGFR compared to the control arm. A significant reduction in MMP-7 and PCX levels, markers of diabetic nephropathy, was observed in the NIC arm [18].

5.3 COVID trials

A Phase 2 randomized clinical trial explored the efficacy of NIC vs. placebo in patients testing positive for SARS-CoV-2 who were either asymptomatic or with mild to moderate COVID-19. The primary efficacy endpoint was the proportion of participants with viral clearance in respiratory samples at day three based on the intention-to-treat (ITT) sample. Secondary endpoints included the proportion of participants with viral clearance in fecal samples at day 14, change in respiratory viral shedding (on days 1, 3, 7, 10, and 14), progression to severe COVID disease, and time to resolution of symptoms reported on day 1. The safety endpoint was defined as the incidence of any adverse event. Patients (73 participants) were randomly assigned to receive either NIC 2 gram (tablet) by mouth daily for 7 days or placebo using the same dosing schedule. NIC was well tolerated without any significant side effects. The efficacy endpoints of oropharyngeal clearance or symptom duration shortening did not significantly differ between the two groups [52].

PROTECT-V, a multicenter randomized controlled trial, aimed to study pre-exposure prophylactic effects of intranasal NIC, nasal and inhaled ciclesonide, or intravenous sotrovimab compared to the matched placebo control groups against SARS-CoV-2 infection for 36 weeks (total 1653 patients) in vulnerable patient populations (organ transplant patients, patients with oncological/hematological diagnoses, immune deficiency or autoimmune diseases requiring immunosuppression or on dialysis). The primary outcomes for the study were confirmed SARS-CoV-2 and one or more COVID-19 symptoms including respiratory, constitutional, or gastrointestinal. The secondary outcomes included (1) time to confirmed SARS-CoV-2 infection, (2) safety and all-cause mortality, and (3) severity of COVID-19 disease. For the NIC arm, the drug was administered as 1% NIC ethanolamine solution and a total daily dose of 5.6 mg NIC ethanolamine salt (4.7 mg free NIC acid) to maximize delivery of the drug to the nasal and upper respiratory tract epithelia. The study did not meet its primary endpoint as no difference was detected between the risk of infection in the NIC and placebo groups. No major safety signals were reported [53].

5.4 Rheumatoid disease

The therapeutic efficacy of NIC in patients was explored in a randomized, double-blind, placebo-controlled trial comparing orally administered NIC (1000 mg once daily) to placebo (lactose) with adjuvant etanercept. All enrolled patients (n = 110) had been on etanercept for more than 3 months prior to enrollment with continued high or moderate active RA. The study assessed the clinical efficacy of NIC using several RA disease activity indices (DAS28, SDAI, CDAI, HAQ-DI). RA markers including changes in erythrocyte sedimentation rate (ESR), C-reactive protein (CRP), levels of IL-1β, IL-6, TNF-α, intercellular adhesion molecule-1 (ICAM-1), vascular adhesion molecule (VCAM-1), and E-selectin were assessed as well. The treatment duration was 60 days. The trial noted significant improvement in RA disease indices in the NIC group with etanercept compared to the placebo with etanercept group. NIC significantly lowered E-selectin, ICAM1, and VCAM1 compared to baseline values. Interestingly, however, unlike the group's aforementioned pre-clinical study, a significant reduction in other inflammatory markers like TNF-2β and IL-1β was not noted [54].

6. Niclosamide repurposing clinical trials summary

(see **Table 1**)

	Clinical trial (NCT#)	Phase and type	Study population and size (n)	Intervention	Primary outcome measure(s)	Study status	Findings summary	Reference
Cancer								
Prostate cancer								
Recurrent or Metastatic castration resistant prostate cancer (CRPC)	NCT03123978	1	Adults (≥19 years old) Enrolled: 6	Niclosamide / PDMX001 oral capsules twice daily (BID) with enzalutamide	Safety and determine RP2D of niclosamide/ (PDMX1001) and enzalutamide	Completed	Results not available	Not published
Metastatic castration resistant prostate cancer (CRPC)	NCT02807805	1b	Adults (≥19 years old) Enrolled: 37	Niclosamide / PDMX1001) oral capsules in escalating dose level frequency (once daily, BID and three times daily (TID) with abiretarone and prednisone	Safety and determine MTD and RP2D of niclosamide/ PDMX1001	Active (not recruiting)	RP2D: 1200 mg PO TID Combination was well tolerated with most frequent adverse effect of diarrhea.	[49]
Metastatic castration resistance prostrate cancer	NCT02532114	1	Adults (≥ 18 years old) Enrolled: 5	Niclosamide (oral) (TID) with enzalutamide (niclosamide formulation not specified)	Safety and determine MTD and RP2D of niclosamide	Terminated	Dose limiting toxicity with 1000 mg TID dosing. Study terminated early due to subtherapeutic niclosamide plasma concentrations at 500 mg TID.	[50]
Colorectal cancer								
Metastatic colorectal cancer (NIKOLO)	NCT02519582	2	Adults (≥ 18 years old) Enrolled: 37	Niclosamide 2 gm tablets (oral) daily	Progression free survival (PFS) at 4 months	Unknown	Results not available	[28]

	Clinical trial (NCT#)	Phase and type	Study population and size (n)	Intervention	Primary outcome measure(s)	Study status	Findings summary	Reference
Pediatric AML (relapsed/ refractory)	NCT05188170	1	Pediatrics and young adults (≥ 2–25 years) Enrolled: Ongoing	Niclosamide capsules (oral) with cytarabine	Safety – determine RP2D of niclosamide	Recruiting	Ongoing	[51]
Metabolic diseases								
Diabetic nephropathy	NCT04317430	3 Randomized Controlled Trial	Adults (≥ 18 years old to 80 years) Enrolled: 82	Niclosamide 1 gm oral tablet daily with ramipril vs. ramipril only	Changes in urinary albumin to creatinine ratio, serum creatinine and estimated glomerular filtrate (eGFR)	Completed	Significant reduction in urinary albumin to creatinine ratio (UACR). Non-significant change in serum creatinine and eGFR	[18]
Autoimmune diseases								
Rheumatoid arthritis	NCT03160001	2 Randomized Double Blind Placebo Controlled Trial	Adults (≥ 18 years old) Enrolled: 110	Niclosamide 500 mg oral capsule twice daily with etanercept vs. placebo (lactose) with etanercept (duration 8 weeks)	Change in Disease Activity Scale/Index	Completed	Significant change noted in disease activity index. Compared to placebo. No significant reduction observed in inflammatory markers such as ESR, CRP, IL-6, TNF-α, IL-1β	[54]

	Clinical trial (NCT#)	Phase and type	Study population and size (n)	Intervention	Primary outcome measure(s)	Study status	Findings summary	Reference
Infectious diseases								
SARS-CoV2 Mild to moderate COVID19	NCT04399356	2 Randomized double blind placebo controlled trial	Adults (≥ 18 years) Enrolled: 73	Niclosamide 2 gm orally daily X 7 days vs. placebo	Time to Respiratory Viral Clearance	Completed	No significant difference in oropharyngeal clearance of SARS-CoV-2 observed between niclosamide and placebo groups	[52]
SARS-CoV2 Prophylaxis in patients at risk of COVID-19 (PROTECT-V)	NCT04870333	2/3 Randomized double blind placebo controlled trial	Adults (≥ 18 years at-risk / vulnerable population) Enrolled: 1653	Intranasal niclosamide and matched placebo	Risk of confirmed and symptomatic SARS-CoV2 (respiratory, constitutional or gastrointestinal symptoms)	Completed	No difference detected between niclosamide and placebo groups	[53]

Table 1.
Niclosamide repurposing clinical trials.

7. Newer formulations

The recent pace of scientific inquiry into novel clinical applications of NIC has surprisingly not been tempered by the limited bioavailability of the agent. This repurposing interest has spurred the scientific community to explore alternative formulations of NIC to comprehensively study and harness its therapeutic potential. Efforts are underway to design oral formulations of NIC with improved solubility and bioavailability compared to the ones currently available, in addition to non-oral formulations, which can yield targeted levels of drug exposure with limited or minimal off-target adverse effects.

In pharmaceutics, various techniques are used for the enhancement of the solubility of poorly soluble drugs which include physical and chemical modifications of drugs and other methods like particle size reduction, crystal engineering, salt formation, solid dispersion, use of surfactant, complexation, etc. [55] An application of some of these methods is evident in the development of an amorphous solid dispersion (ASD) of NIC in an enteric-coated tablet form by Jara and colleagues. The enteric-coated tablets were found to protect the formulation from acidic conditions and prevent polymer gelling. The formulation generated amorphous nanoparticles during dissolution, increasing the drug's solubility from 6.6 mcg/mL to 481 mcg/mL (~70 fold in simulated intestinal fluid) and its bioavailability by 2.6 fold in rats. The study also noted a relatively higher plasma concentration (~150 ng/mL) of NIC when administered at a dose of 75 mg/kg as enteric-coated ASD tablets to beagle dogs compared to that previously reported in the literature for 100 mg/kg solubilized NIC [56]. Further *in vivo* and clinical studies are planned for this novel oral formulation. Another group recently published data on their lipid-based self-micro-emulsifying drug delivery system for NIC (Nic-SMEDDS) [57]. SMEDDS formulation system consists of the drug dissolved or suspended in an oil phase along with a surfactant and a co-surfactant or solubilizer [58]. It creates a greatly enhanced interfacial area, which allows for the easy partition of the drug from the oil phase into the aqueous phase. Yi and colleagues reported a higher Cmax with Nic-SMEDDS (495.3ng/mL) compared to NIC (273ng/mL) and NIC ethanolamine salt (NEN) (346.7ng/mL) following an oral gavage of 40mg/kg dose molecular weight equivalent to NEN. Anti-tumor efficacy in their hepatocellular carcinoma PDX mouse model was also superior for Nic-SMEEDS (100 mg/kg BID) compared to NEN (200 mg/kg once daily) as evidenced by increased levels of Caspase 3 protein and reduced Ki-67 levels. Further pre-clinical and clinical studies utilizing this formulation in other disease models should be explored.

Until now, although alternative more potent and bioavailable oral formulations of NIC, such as O-Alkylamino tethered derivatives, have been reported, their use in the clinic has not been reported [59].

Given the pleiotropic pharmacology of NIC, formulations better suited to the treatment site of interest are also in development. One such example is the intranasal NIC spray, allowing for its local delivery to the site of infection for COVID 19 and other respiratory infections. Union Therapeutics completed Phase 1 testing of their intranasal spray in healthy volunteers, and it was subsequently selected for the PROTECT-V study discussed above [53]. Another group has published research on extraction of NIC from the commercially available NIC tablets and formulating it into throat and nasal sprays as potential therapies for COVID19 and other respiratory viruses including Influenza and Respiratory Syncytial Virus (RSV) [60]. Further testing of this formulation in the clinical realm is currently pending. Besides, throat and nasal sprays, a topical formulation of niclosamide has also been explored. A randomized Phase 2 trial by Weiss and colleagues reported on the use of topical NIC (AT X 201) where it reduced *Staphylococcus aureus* colonization in patients with mild to moderate atopic dermatitis [61].

Intravenous administration of NIC is limited by its low solubility and need for high administration concentration. Re-formulation efforts that can improve its pharmacologic properties including improved solubility and slow release may help overcome these barriers to clinical use. One such approach has been to package NIC in a nanoparticle formulation. A study by Gan and colleagues observed that the intravenously administered nanoparticle formulation of NIC improved both the solubility of the drug and demonstrated in vivo activity for inhibiting and reversing established pulmonary fibrosis [62]. Another group tested intravenous delivery of NIC stearate prodrug therapeutic (NSPT), a nanoparticle formulation of NIC in the lung metastatic mouse model of osteosarcoma [63]. They reported reductions in the metastatic burden as well as improved survival in mice. In addition, the concentrations achieved in the mice after IV NSPT were higher than those achieved after oral dosing of NIC in the phase 1 clinical trial in patients with prostate cancer (dose 0.5 g or 1 g/day) and phase II clinical trial in patients with metastatic colorectal cancer (mCRC) (dose 2 g/day). For example, the median C_{max} of oral NIC was 0.665 mcg/mL (~2 μmol/L) after a 2 g oral dose in patients with mCRC compared to ~70 mcg/mL (~ 210 μmol/L) after NSPT 50 mg/kg (27 mg/kg NIC equivalent) IV dose in mice. Further examination of the safety and efficacy of this IV formulation in animal models and clinical trials is planned.

In recent decades, liposomes have become a key player in the armamentarium of drug formulations. Their therapeutic potential as carriers of drug payloads coupled with a design allowing for delivery of pharmaceuticals to the target site renders them an especially attractive drug formulation for oncologic indications. Their passive (Enhanced Permeability and Retention (EPR) exploiting the leaky nature of tumor-associated blood vessels) and/or active targeting (conjugating to targeting moieties) properties could potentially minimize off-target effects [64]. Hatamipour and colleagues published their experience using NIC nano-liposomes in an experimental model of colon carcinoma. They noted that nano-liposomal NIC showed a higher growth inhibitory activity against the colon carcinoma cells compared to free NIC [65].

Further studies assessing the safety and efficacy signals of this formulation in other disease models are required. With promising results, nano-liposomal encapsulation of NIC could serve as a catalyst in the quest for successfully repurposing NIC. Additionally, more cost effective NIC nano-formulations using FDA-approved excipients are also being tested in the pre-clinical setting along with delivery systems utilizing pegylated NIC [56].

8. NIC drug combinations

Another active area of interest seeks to selectively pair NIC with other drugs in order to potentiate the effect of the combined regimen. This is especially evident in the field of oncology with the goal of maximizing therapeutic efficacy using synergizing or additive drug agents while minimizing adverse effects. Luo F. and colleagues reported findings on their pre-clinical study of combining NIC with PD-1/PDL-1 immune checkpoint inhibitors in NSCLC cell lines and mouse models [66].

The group observed that NIC enhanced the cancer cell lysis mediated by T cells in the presence of PD-L1 blockade. The mice treated with NIC and PD-L1 antibody showed significant delay in tumor growth and increased survival, which were associated with the increase of tumor infiltrating T cells and granzyme B release. An enhancement of PD-L1 antibody by NIC was observed in the inhibition of non-small cell lung cancer (NSCLC) growth *in vitro* and *in vivo*, which was involved in the blockage of p-STAT3 binding to the promoter of PD-L1 and finally downregulation of PD-L1 expression. Given its inhibitory effect on the STAT3 pathway, NIC may also help attenuate drug resistance to epidermal growth factor inhibitor receptor inhibitors (EGFRi) induced by activation of STAT3 by EGFRi [67]. This was demonstrated in findings by Li and colleagues where NIC in combination with erlotinib potently repressed erlotinib-resistant lung cancer xenografts in association with increased apoptosis in tumor tissues, suggesting that NIC could restore sensitivity to erlotinib [68]. Chae H and colleagues reported NIC synergizing with acute myeloid leukemia (AML) first-line chemotherapy drug cytarabine by inhibiting the CREB-dependent pathway and NF-κB pathway and increasing reactive oxygen species (ROS) levels [35]. This combination is currently being investigated in a pediatric AML clinical trial by Sakamoto et al. [51]. Due to the extensive network of signaling pathways targeted by NIC, many other chemotherapeutic agents and targeted therapies could synergize with NIC [67]. An optimization of NIC formulation allowing for enhanced bioavailability would greatly assist in accelerating this area of research.

9. Conclusions

NIC has demonstrated significant potential as a multi-target therapeutic agent in pre-clinical high-throughput bioassays and mouse model studies. As highlighted in this chapter, a limiting factor toward fully harnessing the therapeutic potential of NIC has been the achievement of drug exposures needed for effect outside the gastrointestinal tract due to its poor oral bioavailability and limited ability to be given intravenously. This limitation has led to the exploration of newer formulations of NIC with optimized pharmaceutics and improved pharmacokinetics of the agent. However, additional studies of these newer formulations are required to better elucidate the safety of NIC at systemic exposures required for effects outside the gastrointestinal tract. The potential applicability would need to be carefully calibrated against adverse effects potentially resulting from its multi-receptor targeting. A further refinement of the aforementioned formulation designs and/or coupling them with a more targeted approach could position NIC as a promising therapeutic agent, particularly with regard to oncologic indications. One such measure could be a drug antibody conjugate, which would link the specificity of a monoclonal antibody to NIC's cytotoxic payload. Additionally, a drug-monoclonal antibody conjugate fashioned as a liposomal nanoparticle designed to deploy both passive (EPR) and active targeting strategies for a tumor-specific targeting could potentially be an even more effective approach. A deeper exploration of NIC pharmacology, molecular modeling, and signaling targets is necessitated to transform the underutilized potential of this agent into a viable therapeutic.

Although several clinical trials have been conducted for cancer (AML, prostate, colorectal), COVID, diabetic nephropathy, and rheumatoid arthritis, the exact dose, frequency, and indications have yet to be determined. Niclosamide is generally well-tolerated. Nevertheless, in the clinical trial with prostate cancer in elderly men, the optimal phase 2 dose was not obtainable at the highest doses due to toxicity and poor oral availability. Furthermore, the plasma concentrations at the maximum tolerated dose were not consistently above the desired therapeutic threshold [50]. While this may be true for the other ongoing clinical trials, the studies are too early to make any conclusions. In summary, there are many potential indications for repurposing NIC based on pre-clinical studies, however, additional information is needed to determine which disease would be ideal for future clinical trials.

Acknowledgements

We would like to acknowledge the Leukemia & Lymphoma Society (K.M.S. and N.L.) and the Pediatric Cancer Research Foundation (K.M.S) for their support.

Conflict of interest

The authors declare no conflict of interest.

Author details

Namrata Patel[1*†], Kailen Mark[2†], Adam Frymoyer[3], Norman Lacayo[2] and Kathleen M. Sakamoto[2]

1 Department of Pharmacy, Lucile Packard Children's Hospital, Palo Alto, CA, USA

2 Department of Pediatrics, Stanford Cancer Institute, Stanford University School of Medicine, Stanford, CA, USA

3 Department of Neonatal and Developmental Medicine, Stanford School of Medicine, Stanford, CA, USA

*Address all correspondence to: napatel@stanfordchildrens.org

† Co-first authors.

References

[1] Weinbach EC, Garbus J. Mechanism of action of reagents that uncouple oxidative phosphorylation. Nature. 1969;**221**(5185):1016-1018

[2] Alasadi A, Chen M, Swapna GVT, et al. Effect of mitochondrial uncouplers niclosamide ethanolamine (NEN) and oxyclozanide on hepatic metastasis of colon cancer. Cell Death & Disease. 2018;**9**(2):215

[3] Chen W, Mook RA Jr, Premont RT, Wang J. Niclosamide: Beyond an antihelminthic drug. Cellular Signalling. 2018;**41**:89-96

[4] Jara M. The challenge of repurposing niclosamide: Considering pharmacokinetic parameters, routes of administration, and drug metabolism. Journal of Drug Delivery Science and Technology. 2023;**81**:104187

[5] Singh S, Weiss A, Goodman J, et al. Niclosamide-A promising treatment for COVID-19. British Journal of Pharmacology. 2022;**179**(13):3250-3267

[6] Kumar R, Coronel L, Somalanka B, et al. Mitochondrial uncoupling reveals a novel therapeutic opportunity for p53-defective cancers. Nature Communications. 2018;**9**(1):3931

[7] Andrews P, Thyssen J, Lorke D. The biology and toxicology of molluscicides, bayluscide. Pharmacology & Therapeutics. 1982;**19**(2):245-295

[8] Biersack B. The antifungal potential of niclosamide and structurally related salicylanilides. International Journal of Molecular Sciences. 2024;**25**(11):1-21

[9] Hamdoun S, Jung P, Efferth T. Drug repurposing of the anthelmintic niclosamide to treat multidrug-resistant leukemia. Frontiers in Pharmacology. 2017;**8**:110

[10] Braga L, Ali H, Secco I, et al. Drugs that inhibit TMEM16 proteins block SARS-CoV-2 spike-induced syncytia. Nature. 2021;**594**(7861):88-93

[11] Vazquez-Rodriguez JA, Shaqour B, Guarch-Perez C, et al. A Niclosamide-releasing hot-melt extruded catheter prevents Staphylococcus aureus experimental biomaterial-associated infection. Scientific Reports. 2022;**12**(1):12329

[12] Rajamuthiah R, Fuchs BB, Conery AL, et al. Repurposing salicylanilide anthelmintic drugs to combat drug resistant Staphylococcus aureus. PLoS One. 2015;**10**(4):e0124595

[13] Sutar Y, Nabeela S, Singh S, et al. Niclosamide-loaded nanoparticles disrupt Candida biofilms and protect mice from mucosal candidiasis. PLoS Biology. 2022;**20**(8):e3001762

[14] Cabrita I, Benedetto R, Schreiber R, Kunzelmann K. Niclosamide repurposed for the treatment of inflammatory airway disease. JCI Insight. 2019;**4**(15):1-15

[15] Liang L, Huang M, Xiao Y, et al. Inhibitory effects of niclosamide on inflammation and migration of fibroblast-like synoviocytes from patients with rheumatoid arthritis. Inflammation Research. 2015;**64**(3-4):225-233

[16] Al-Gareeb A, Gorial F, Mahmood A. The anti-rheumatoid activity of niclosamide in collagen-induced arthritis in rats. Archives of Rheumatology. 2019;**34**(4):426-433

[17] Tao H, Zhang Y, Zeng X, Shulman GI, Jin S. Niclosamide ethanolamine-induced mild mitochondrial uncoupling improves diabetic symptoms in mice. Nature Medicine. 2014;**20**(11):1263-1269

[18] El-Fatatry BM, El-Haggar SM, Ibrahim OM, Shalaby KH. Niclosamide from an anthelmintic drug to a promising adjuvant therapy for diabetic kidney disease: Randomized clinical trial. Diabetology and Metabolic Syndrome. 2023;**15**(1):22

[19] Chang X, Zhen X, Liu J, et al. The antihelmenthic phosphate niclosamide impedes renal fibrosis by inhibiting homeodomain-interacting protein kinase 2 expression. Kidney International. 2017;**92**(3):612-624

[20] Zhang LX, Zhao HJ, Sun DL, Gao SL, Zhang HM, Ding XG. Niclosamide attenuates inflammatory cytokines via the autophagy pathway leading to improved outcomes in renal ischemia/reperfusion injury. Molecular Medicine Reports. 2017;**16**(2):1810-1816

[21] Chen Q, Gao C, Wang M, Fei X, Zhao N. TRIM18-regulated STAT3 signaling pathway via PTP1B promotes renal epithelial-mesenchymal transition, inflammation, and fibrosis in diabetic kidney disease. Frontiers in Physiology. 2021;**12**:709506

[22] Li Y, Li P, He Q, et al. Niclosamide inhibits hepatitis E virus through suppression of NF-kappaB signalling. Antiviral Research. 2022;**197**:105228

[23] Xu J, Xue Y, Bolinger AA, et al. Therapeutic potential of salicylamide derivatives for combating viral infections. Medicinal Research Reviews. 2023;**43**(4):897-931

[24] Fu Y, Hu N, Cao M, et al. Anthelmintic niclosamide attenuates pressure-overload induced heart failure in mice. European Journal of Pharmacology. 2021;**912**:174614

[25] Li SL, Yan J, Zhang YQ, et al. Niclosamide ethanolamine inhibits artery constriction. Pharmacological Research. 2017;**115**:78-86

[26] Engin S, Yasar YK, Barut EN, Sezen SF. Improved endothelium-dependent relaxation of thoracic aorta in niclosamide-treated diabetic rats. Cardiovascular Toxicology. 2021;**21**(7):563-571

[27] Osada T, Chen M, Yang XY, et al. Antihelminth compound niclosamide downregulates Wnt signaling and elicits antitumor responses in tumors with activating APC mutations. Cancer Research. 2011;**71**(12):4172-4182

[28] Burock S, Daum S, Keilholz U, Neumann K, Walther W, Stein U. Phase II trial to investigate the safety and efficacy of orally applied niclosamide in patients with metachronous or sychronous metastases of a colorectal cancer progressing after therapy: The NIKOLO trial. BMC Cancer. 2018;**18**(1):297

[29] Yu X, Liu F, Zeng L, et al. Niclosamide exhibits potent anticancer activity and synergizes with sorafenib in human renal cell cancer cells. Cellular Physiology and Biochemistry. 2018;**47**(3):957-971

[30] He Y, Luo Y, Huang L, et al. New frontiers against sorafenib resistance in renal cell carcinoma: From molecular mechanisms to predictive biomarkers. Pharmacological Research. 2021;**170**:105732

[31] Yun JM, Woo SM, Seo SU, Min KJ, Kim DE, Kwon TK. Involvement of up-regulation of DR5 expression and down-regulation of c-FLIP

in niclosamide-mediated TRAIL sensitization in human renal carcinoma caki cells. Molecules. 2018;**23**(9):1-11

[32] Liu C, Lou W, Armstrong C, Zhu Y, Evans CP, Gao AC. Niclosamide suppresses cell migration and invasion in enzalutamide resistant prostate cancer cells via Stat3-AR axis inhibition. Prostate. 2015;**75**(13):1341-1353

[33] Jiang H, Li AM, Ye J. The magic bullet: Niclosamide. Frontiers in Oncology. 2022;**12**:1004978

[34] Jin Y, Lu Z, Ding K, et al. Antineoplastic mechanisms of niclosamide in acute myelogenous leukemia stem cells: Inactivation of the NF-κB pathway and generation of reactive oxygen species. Cancer Research. 2010;**70**(6):2516-2527

[35] Chae HD, Cox N, Dahl GV, et al. Niclosamide suppresses acute myeloid leukemia cell proliferation through inhibition of CREB-dependent signaling pathways. Oncotarget. 2018;**9**(4):4301-4317

[36] Kantarjian H, Kadia T, DiNardo C, et al. Acute myeloid leukemia: Current progress and future directions. Blood Cancer Journal. 2021;**11**(2):41

[37] Shimony S, Stahl M, Stone RM. Acute myeloid leukemia: 2023 update on diagnosis, risk-stratification, and management. American Journal of Hematology. 2023;**98**(3):502-526

[38] Mesbahi Y, Trahair TN, Lock RB, Connerty P. Exploring the metabolic landscape of AML: From haematopoietic stem cells to myeloblasts and leukaemic stem cells. Frontiers in Oncology. 2022;**12**:807266

[39] Farge T, Saland E, de Toni F, et al. Chemotherapy-resistant human acute myeloid leukemia cells are not enriched for leukemic stem cells but require oxidative metabolism. Cancer Discovery. 2017;**7**(7):716-735

[40] Satoh K, Zhang L, Zhang Y, et al. Identification of niclosamide as a novel anticancer agent for adrenocortical carcinoma. Clinical Cancer Research. 2016;**22**(14):3458-3466

[41] Yo Y-T, Lin Y-W, Wang Y-C, et al. Growth inhibition of ovarian tumor–initiating cells by niclosamide. Molecular Cancer Therapeutics. 2012;**11**(8):1703-1712

[42] Park SJ, Shin JH, Kang H, Hwang JJ, Cho DH. Niclosamide induces mitochondria fragmentation and promotes both apoptotic and autophagic cell death. BMB Reports. 2011;**44**(8):517-522

[43] Cheng JC, Kinjo K, Judelson DR, et al. CREB is a critical regulator of normal hematopoiesis and leukemogenesis. Blood. 2008;**111**(3):1182-1192

[44] Shankar DB, Cheng JC, Kinjo K, et al. The role of CREB as a proto-oncogene in hematopoiesis and in acute myeloid leukemia. Cancer Cell. 2005;**7**(4):351-362

[45] Mayr B, Montminy M. Transcriptional regulation by the phosphorylation-dependent factor CREB. Nature Reviews Molecular Cell Biology. 2001;**2**(8):599-609

[46] Best JL, Amezcua CA, Mayr B, et al. Identification of small-molecule antagonists that inhibit an activator: Coactivator interaction. Proceedings of the National Academy of Sciences of the United States of America. 2004;**101**(51):17622-17627

[47] Mitton B, Chae HD, Hsu K, et al. Small molecule inhibition of cAMP

response element binding protein in human acute myeloid leukemia cells. Leukemia. 2016;**30**(12):2302-2311

[48] Chae HD, Cox N, Capolicchio S, et al. SAR optimization studies on modified salicylamides as a potential treatment for acute myeloid leukemia through inhibition of the CREB pathway. Bioorganic & Medicinal Chemistry Letters. 2019;**29**(16):2307-2315

[49] Parikh M, Liu C, Wu CY, et al. Phase Ib trial of reformulated niclosamide with abiraterone/prednisone in men with castration-resistant prostate cancer. Scientific Reports. 2021;**11**(1):6377

[50] Schweizer MT, Haugk K, McKiernan JS, et al. A phase I study of niclosamide in combination with enzalutamide in men with castration-resistant prostate cancer. PLoS One. 2018;**13**(6):e0198389

[51] Sakamoto KM. Niclosamide in Pediatric Patients and Young Adults with Relapsed and Refractory AML. clinicaltrialsgov; 2022. Available from: https://clinicaltrials.gov

[52] Caims DM. Efficacy of niclosamide vs. placebo in SARS-CoV-2 respiratory viral clearance, viral shedding, and duration of symptoms among patients with mild to moderate COVID-19 - A phase 2 randomized clinical trial. JAMA Network Open. 2022;**5**(2):2144942

[53] Humphrey TJL, Dosanjh D, Hiemstra TF, et al. Prophylaxis for patients at risk of COVID-19 infection (PROTECT-V). Trials. 2023;**24**(1):185

[54] Al-Gareeb AIA, Gorial FI, Mahmood AS. Niclosamide as an adjuvant to etanercept in treatment patients with active rheumatoid arthritis: An 8-week randomized controlled pilot study. Clinical Rheumatology. 2018;**37**(10):2633-2641

[55] Savjani KT, Gajjar AK, Savjani JK. Drug solubility: Importance and enhancement techniques. ISRN Pharmacology. 2012;**2012**:195727

[56] Jara MO, Warnken ZN, Sahakijpijarn S, et al. Oral delivery of niclosamide as an amorphous solid dispersion that generates amorphous nanoparticles during dissolution. Pharmaceutics. 2022;**14**(12):1-14

[57] Liu Q, Zhang Q, Yao Z, et al. Pushing forward the DNA walkers in connection with tumor-derived extracellular vesicles. International Journal of Nanomedicine. 2024;**19**:6231-6252

[58] Shah AK, Agnihotri SA. Recent advances and novel strategies in pre-clinical formulation development: An overview. Journal of Controlled Release. 2011;**156**(3):281-296

[59] Chen H, Yang Z, Ding C, et al. Discovery of O-alkylamino tethered niclosamide derivatives as potent and orally bioavailable anticancer agents. ACS Medicinal Chemistry Letters. 2013;**4**(2):180-185

[60] Needham D. Extraction of niclosamide from commercial approved tablets into aqueous buffered solution creates potentially approvable oral and nasal sprays against COVID-19 and other respiratory infections. AAPS Open. 2023;**9**(1):9

[61] Weiss A, Delavenne E, Matias C, et al. Topical niclosamide (ATx201) reduces Staphylococcus aureus colonization and increases Shannon diversity of the skin microbiome in atopic dermatitis patients in a randomized, double-blind, placebo-controlled phase 2 trial. Clinical and Translational Medicine. 2022;**12**(5):e790

[62] Gan C, Wang Y, Xiang Z, et al. Niclosamide-loaded nanoparticles (Ncl-NPs) reverse pulmonary fibrosis in vivo and in vitro. Journal of Advanced Research. 2023;**51**:109-120

[63] Reddy GB, Kerr DL, Spasojevic I, et al. Preclinical testing of a novel niclosamide stearate prodrug therapeutic (NSPT) shows efficacy against osteosarcoma. Molecular Cancer Therapeutics. 2020;**19**(7):1448-1461

[64] Deshpande PP, Biswas S, Torchilin VP. Current trends in the use of liposomes for tumor targeting. Nanomedicine (London, England). 2013;**8**(9):1509-1528

[65] Hatamipour M, Jaafari MR, Momtazi-Borojeni AA, Ramezani M, Sahebkar A. Evaluation of the anti-tumor activity of niclosamide nanoliposomes against colon carcinoma. Current Molecular Pharmacology. 2020;**13**(3):245-250

[66] Luo F, Luo M, Rong QX, et al. Niclosamide, an antihelmintic drug, enhances efficacy of PD-1/PD-L1 immune checkpoint blockade in non-small cell lung cancer. Journal for Immunotherapy of Cancer. 2019;**7**(1):245

[67] Ren J, Wang B, Wu Q, Wang G. Combination of niclosamide and current therapies to overcome resistance for cancer: New frontiers for an old drug. Biomedicine & Pharmacotherapy. 2022;**155**:113789

[68] Li R, Hu Z, Sun SY, et al. Niclosamide overcomes acquired resistance to erlotinib through suppression of STAT3 in non-small cell lung cancer. Molecular Cancer Therapeutics. 2013;**12**(10):2200-2212

Chapter 7

Unlocking Brigatinib's Potential: A Remarkable Case of Drug Repurposing in NF2-SWN

Annette Bakker, D. Wade Clapp, James Gusella, Jaishri Blakeley, Scott Plotkin and Marc Ferrer

Abstract

Synodos for NF2 is a collaborative research initiative aimed at accelerating the development of treatments for NF2-related schwannomatosis, a complex and rare genetic disorder. Leveraging resources like the National Center for Advancing Translational Sciences drug screening platform with the MIPE oncology collection, the team identified Brigatinib, an unexpected hit, as a potential therapeutic agent. Through subsequent proteomics analysis, Focal Adhesion Kinase was identified as the primary target of Brigatinib, revealing a novel mechanism of action for the drug in NF2-related schwannomatosis. This discovery led to the development of the Innovative Trial for Understanding the Impact of Targeted Therapies in NF2-Related Schwannomatosis platform-basket trial, which rapidly translated these findings into a clinical trial framework. Preliminary results from this trial have shown promising efficacy, marking a significant step forward in NF2-related schwannomatosis treatment. The collaborative efforts of Synodos and the innovative platform trial approach are paving the way for more efficient drug discovery and development in NF2-related schwannomatosis, offering new hope for patients with this challenging disorder.

Keywords: Brigatinib, NF2-related schwannomatosis, platform-basket trial, drug repurposing, synodos collaborative

1. Introduction

1.1 NF2-related Schwannomatosis

NF2-related schwannomatosis (NF2-SWN) is a rare genetic disorder with a prevalence of 1 in 55,000 individuals globally [1]. First described in the early twentieth century, NF2-SWN is a progressive multi-organ disorder characterized by the formation of multiple benign tumors along the nerves, affecting the central and peripheral nervous systems. The hallmark tumor of the disease is the development of bilateral vestibular schwannomas, tumors that occur on the 8th cranial nerve. The tumors often lead to hearing loss and balance issues. In addition to vestibular schwannomas, individuals with NF2-SWN may develop other types of tumors, such as meningiomas, ependymomas, and non-vestibular schwannomas [2, 3].

NF2-SWN is caused by germline pathogenic variants in the NF2 gene located on chromosome 22 [4]. This gene encodes the tumor suppressor protein Merlin (moesin–ezrin–radixin-like), a crucial regulator of cell growth and maintenance of cellular architecture. Loss of Merlin function in NF2-SWN disrupts normal cell signaling pathways, leading to uncontrolled cell proliferation and benign tumor formation [5].

1.2 Complexity of the NF2 gene/Merlin downstream pathways

Merlin, a member of the Ezrin, Radixin, and Moesin (ERM) family, acts as a tumor suppressor by inhibiting several oncogenic signaling pathways, including cell proliferation, migration, and survival. Merlin regulates signaling pathways mostly by direct interaction through its FERM domain and C-terminal tail. These interactions occur with several binding partners involved in the same pathway, reinforcing Merlin's control of the pathway at several levels, for example, Hippo pathway modulation occurs via Merlin's interaction with LATS1/2, angiomotin (AMOT), E3 ubiquitin ligase CRL4-DCAF1, and TEAD4 [6]. Therefore, targeting a pathway must take into consideration all the levels of Merlin involvement and ensure that the downstream elements are also influenced by the drug. In addition, signaling pathway crosstalk can be cell type-specific, and combining targets should be adapted to the tumor type.

The intricate role of Merlin in various signaling pathways makes treating NF2-SWN challenging. Although all tumors in NF2-SWN patients exhibit Merlin loss, their responses to treatment can vary significantly due to differences in expression profiles [7]. This variability may suggest that effective treatment might require a combination of multiple therapeutic agents. However, managing such a complex treatment regimen is particularly difficult given the chronic nature of the condition, which necessitates long-term treatment.

1.3 Target and treatment opportunities in NF2-SWN

Research has identified two main treatment opportunities in NF2-SWN: (1) those that will specifically affect the tumor cells and (2) those that could impact the tumor microenvironment. Although the list of signaling pathways in NF2-SWN is constantly growing, the main signaling pathways that are dysregulated and have led to clinical trials in these tumors are:

- *Epidermal Growth Factor Receptor (EGFR) Pathway*: EGFR inhibitors, such as lapatinib and icotinib [8], have shown promise in preclinical studies, but the clinical response has been quite variable across the different NF2-SWN tumor types [9].

- *Akt/mTOR pathway*: mTORC1 inhibitors such as Rapamycin and Everolimus have demonstrated efficacy in the NF2-SWN preclinical models [10], but it is unclear whether they are efficacious in a clinical setting. mTOR inhibitors have shown a cytostatic effect resulting in tumor stasis, but unless there is inhibition of both mTOR complexes (C1/C2), no chemotoxic effect was observed [11]. PI-3 k inhibitors such as CUDC907 have shown *in vitro* [12] but unclear *in vivo* activity preclinically.

- *Hippo/YAP Pathway*: Extensive preclinical work demonstrated that the Hippo pathway activation plays an important role in NF2-SWN tumor development [13, 14]. Some Hippo/YAP pathway inhibitors are undergoing phase 1 evaluation (NCT04665206).

- *HDAC Pathway*: Some HDAC inhibitors (Panobinostat, Vorinostat, AR42) have emerged as potential therapies for NF2-SWN. AR-42 (also known as also known as REC-2282 or OSU-HDAC42) is an orally bioavailable pan-histone deacetylase inhibitor currently in efficacy trial for meningioma [15, 16].

- *VEGF Pathway*: Bevacizumab is an anti-VEGF antibody that affects the tumor microenvironment, is used in a clinical setting, and has demonstrated improved hearing and tumor reduction in NF2-SWN patients [17].

- *Integrin receptors*: Merlin links actin to transmembrane proteins. Recent work has indicated a potential role for integrin-mediated signals in NF2-SWN, leading to pathological elevation of focal adhesion kinase [18] that in turn signals activation in the Ras-PI3K-MEK-ERk pathway as well as the hippo pathway. Brigatinib, the drug recently found to result in a biological signature in schwannomas and meningiomas and meningiomas is an RTK that inhibits focal adhesion kinase in a dose-dependent fashion [18].

In recent years, research around NF2-SWN tumor microenvironment and treatments that affect fibrosis and inflammation opened novel avenues for combination therapies that affect the tumor and the microenvironment. miRNAs, such as miR-24-3p [19] and miR21 [20], may hold new therapeutic avenues for the NF2-SWN patients.

2. Challenges in NF2-SWN treatment: Tumor heterogeneity

One of the challenges in treating NF2-SWN is the diversity of tumor types and their variable responses to treatment. NF2-SWN encompasses a range of tumors, including vestibular schwannomas, non-vestibular schwannomas, meningiomas, and ependymomas, which may arise within the same patient at the same moment. Each of these tumor types arises from different cell lineages and exhibits different biological behaviors and responses to therapeutic interventions. The complexity of the disease may necessitate a nuanced approach to treatment, including the need for personalized combination therapies.

- *Bilateral Vestibular Schwannomas:* Vestibular schwannomas typically affect the 8th cranial (vestibulocochlear) nerve. They are generally slow-growing but can cause significant morbidity due to their location in the brain. They may induce hearing loss, balance issues, tinnitus, and even brain stem compression. Treatment options include surgical resection and radiation therapy, but these interventions carry substantial risks, including hearing and facial nerve damage. Targeted therapies aimed at the NF2-SWN-specific signaling pathways in vestibular schwannomas have shown mixed results, as referred above, emphasizing the need for more targeted treatment options. Vestibular schwannomas are also characterized by an important inflammatory component [21], which may affect treatment selection.

- *Non-Vestibular Schwannomas:* Although less common, these tumors can occur along any peripheral nerve and may present with different clinical symptoms depending on their location. Non-vestibular schwannomas tend to be more heterogeneous in their biological characteristics, making them challenging to treat.

- *Meningiomas:* Meningiomas benign tumors originating from the arachnoid cap cells. These tumors can induce significant morbidities, including headaches, seizures, and spinal cord compression. Although these tumors reside outside the blood-brain barrier, treatments developed for NF2-SWN patients may also benefit patients with sporadic NF2-negative meningioma.

- *Ependymomas:* Ependymomas arise from ependymal cells lining the brain's ventricles and the spinal cord's central canal. In NF2-SWN patients, ependymomas are relatively rare but can be particularly aggressive. The treatment of ependymomas is challenging due to their location within the spinal cord. Current therapies, including surgery and radiation, are often associated with significant morbidity, and there is a pressing need for more effective systemic therapies.

All tumor types could potentially be treated by surgery. Still, due to the unfavorable consequences of the physical intervention, there is a high unmet medical need for effective and tolerable systemic therapies.

3. Clinical trial design

The diversity and progressive nature of the NF2-SWN tumors pose significant challenges in the design and execution of clinical trials. Moreover, as in all rare diseases, recruiting sufficient clinical trial participants (clinical trial sites and patients) in a reasonable time makes clinical trials in NF2-SWN difficult. The NF2-SWN community has therefore developed:

- *Standardized clinical trial endpoints:* One of the critical challenges in NF2-SWN clinical trials is the standardization of endpoints. Defining meaningful endpoints that can be applied across all patients is problematic due to the diversity of tumor types and their varying growth rates. Moreover, functional outcomes, such as hearing preservation or improved neurological function, may be more relevant than traditional radiographic endpoints. Still, these measures are often more subjective and more challenging to quantify. To build global consensus around standardized endpoints in the NF/SWN community, the Response Evaluation in NF and schwannomatosis International Collaboration (REiNS) was created in 2011. REiNS, comprised of clinicians doing clinical trials, regulatory experts, patients, and industry stakeholders, is organized around nine working groups that all volunteer their time to focus on the following topics: functional outcomes, patient-reported outcomes, visual outcomes, neurocognitive outcomes, imaging outcomes, disease biomarkers, cutaneous neurofibromas, gene therapy, and patient representatives. The consensus papers for REiNS are published in *Neurology* [22, 23].

- *Platform-Basket Trials:* The rarity of NF2-SWN makes patient recruitment for clinical trials particularly challenging. Many patients are treated at specialty centers, and there may be geographic barriers to trial participation. Additionally, the progressive nature of the disease means that patients often undergo multiple treatments over time, which can complicate their eligibility for trials. Innovative trial designs, such as platform-basket trials, may help overcome some of these challenges. Innovative Trial for Understanding the Impact of Targeted Therapies in NF2-Related Schwannomatosis (INTUITT-NF2, NCT04374305) is a multi-arm phase II platform-basket signal-finding screening trial designed to test the radiographic tumor response of multiple experimental therapies simultaneously in patients with NF2-SWN. The Principal Investigator, Dr. Plotkin from MGH, collaborates with seven clinical trial sites (UMiami, JHU, NYU, Mayo, UCLA, IU) to execute the trial while accelerating patient recruitment and improving clinical trial decision-making. The master protocol includes all NF2-SWN patients with progressive vestibular schwannomas, non-vestibular schwannomas, meningiomas, and/or ependymomas. The primary endpoint is radiographic response of target tumors (selected by the treating physician); key secondary endpoints include radiographic response in all tumors, hearing, quality of life, and toxicity. Non-responders to a given drug sub-study will be allowed to be enrolled in a subsequent drug sub-study.

- *Ethical Considerations:* Developing treatments for rare diseases like NF2-SWN involves critical ethical considerations. Although NF2-SWN pathways overlap with oncology pathways, and treatments may be available, patients with NF2-SWN require long-term exposure to drugs often not optimized for prolonged use. This necessitates balancing the exploration of novel therapies with minimizing unnecessary risks to patients. In this context, informed consent as well as patient engagement, is especially important, ensuring that patients fully understand the potential risks and benefits of participating in trials involving experimental treatments with limited long-term safety data. The Children's Tumor Foundation has built an extensive patient engagement initiative (ctf.org/patientengagement).

4. Preclinical model systems

4.1 Cell line models

Cell lines derived from NF2-SWN tumors provide the highest throughput option for studying tumor biology and drug responses. However, cell line models have significant limitations, particularly in their ability to mimic the complex interactions between tumors and their surrounding microenvironment. Furthermore, cell lines, such as HEI193, often undergo genetic and phenotypic changes after extended periods in culture, affecting their relevance to human disease. To address the genetic and phenotypic drift of the commercially available cell lines, multiple groups have generated primary schwannoma [24], meningioma cell lines, and three-dimensional spheroid models [25] for drug screening purposes. Testing the effects of drugs on a panel of cellular models (each with its values and limitations) is critical to assess pharmacological responses based on targets and signaling pathways for better selection of therapeutic assets for preclinical development toward an Investigational New Drug (IND) application, both as single agents or combinations.

4.2 Animal models

Murine models are the most commonly used animal models in NF2-SWN research. The most frequently used transgenic models are the P0Cre Nf2flox2/flox2 [26] and the Postn-Cre; Nf2flox/flox mice [27]. The P0Cre mice develop both benign and malignant Schwann cell tumors later in life (from 10 months on). The Postn-Cre models not only show spinal, peripheral, and cranial nerve tumors, but the development of cranial nerve VIII tumors correlates with functional impairments in hearing and balance, as measured by auditory brainstem response and vestibular testing. The NF2-SWN swine model, in which a premature termination codon in exon 2 of the NF2 gene was introduced, did not result in any NF2-SWN tumors – even after 2 years of observation (unpublished). The NF2-SWN community also developed orthotopic NF2-SWN mouse models by injecting immortalized schwannoma cells, that were stably transduced with fluorescent protein or luciferase reporters, in the sciatic nerve of mice [28] or luciferase-labeled benign meningioma cells in the brain [29]. All *in vivo* model systems have complementary benefits. While the orthotopic models can give quick answers about the effect of an asset on the tumor, the Tg models have an intact (mouse) microenvironment.

4.3 Emerging preclinical models and application to NF2-SWN

Recognizing the limited number of available/accessible preclinical models and tissue samples and the openness of the FDA to consider NMAs (https://www.congress.gov/bill/117th-congress/senate-bill/5002/text, https://www.science.org/content/resource/new-path-new-drugs-finding-alternatives-to-animal-testing) for indications with a high unmet medical need, there is currently an explosion of new models:

- *Advanced Cell Culture Systems:* A range of advanced cellular systems are now being developed to mimic human tissues and organs. These cellular models attempt to capture interactions between different cell types and between cells and the microenvironment and other tissues and organs. Three-dimensional aggregates of cell lines or patient-derived tumors form spheroids-induced [25] pluripotent stem cells (iPSC) can be used to differentiate into organoid models [30, 31]; there are also engineered systems that are bioprinted to include vascularized microenviroment [32, 33] or are developed in tissue chip platforms to include dynamic flow [34]. These models offer a more physiologically relevant environment for studying tumor biology and drug responses compared to traditional two-dimensional cell cultures, as they are expected to reproduce many of the structural and functional characteristics of the original tissue. The NIH is funding the development of NF2-SWN inner ear organoids, which could provide a new model for testing therapies (NIH 2021F30 DC and NIH 2020F30 DC).

- *CRISPR-Cas9 Gene Editing:* CRISPR-Cas9 technology has revolutionized the field of preclinical modeling by enabling precise genetic modifications. This technology will allow the researchers to create more accurate models of NF2-SWN, including models that more closely mimic the human immune system, improving the predictive value of preclinical studies.

5. Need for a comprehensive preclinical platform

5.1 Current translatability limitations

The development of effective therapies has been hindered by (1) the assumption that one preclinical model can recapitulate all aspects of human disease and should be able to predict clinical outcomes and (2) the separation of translational scientists and clinical trialists. The construction of a comprehensive preclinical platform (Synodos NF2), including all stakeholders (basic, translation, clinical scientists, and the patients), with a diverse set of preclinical models – with known limitations and alignment between the preclinical and clinical outcomes has shown to accelerate and improve clinical outcome drastically.

5.1.1 Mixed success of mTOR inhibitors

The mTOR pathway is a central cell growth, proliferation, and survival regulator. In NF2-SWN, mTOR inhibitors have been explored as potential treatments. However, the success of these inhibitors has been inconsistent across different models and clinical trials.

- *mTOR pathway inhibitors in preclinical models:* The mTOR inhibitors, such as everolimus and sirolimus, work by blocking the activity of mTOR C1, thereby inhibiting tumor development in the P0Cre Nf2flox/flox model [35]. While preclinical studies in NF2-SWN models showed promise, with reduced tumor growth and improved survival in mice, the translation of these findings to the clinic has been less successful.

- *Review of clinical trials and their outcomes:* Several clinical trials have investigated the efficacy of mTOR C1 inhibitors in NF2-SWN patients. One of the most notable studies was a phase II trial of everolimus in patients with progressive vestibular schwannomas. While some patients experienced tumor stabilization, the trial failed to meet its primary endpoint defined as ≥15% decrease in vestibular schwannoma volume [36].

- *Hypotheses for why certain models succeeded and others failed:* Several factors may explain the discrepancy between preclinical results and clinical expectations with mTOR inhibitors. In the P0Cre preclinical model, the delay of tumor onset is measured, whereas the clinical trial endpoint requires tumor shrinkage. A collaboration between the translational scientists and the clinicians is essential to allow precise alignment between the preclinical and clinical read-out upfront to improve clinical trial asset selection and clinical outcomes.

5.2 Development of synodos

The Synodos NF2 preclinical platform was aimed at improving the probability of success of treatments in the clinic. The platform was established as a comprehensive, collaborative preclinical testing system for NF2-SWN. This platform brings together researchers, clinicians, and patients to co-design and select treatments ready for clinical trials, utilizing diverse preclinical models and ensuring early alignment of preclinical and clinical outcomes [37].

- *Overview of the creation and collaboration within SYNODOS:* SYNODOS was launched and funded by the Children's Tumor Foundation (CTF) as part of a broader effort to accelerate the development of therapies for NF2-SWN. The global platform was assembled by the NF2-SWN community as a collaboration between multiple research institutions, each contributing unique expertise and resources [37]. One of the critical strengths of SYNODOS is its use of multiple preclinical models to test potential therapies. These models include cell lines (commercial and primary), transgenic animal, and tumor cell-derived orthotopic animal models, each providing unique insights into tumor biology and drug response. By testing drugs across this range of models, SYNODOS was able to identify which therapies are most likely to succeed in the clinic and which ones may need further optimization. Integrated transcriptome, kinome, and proteome data contributed to the basic understanding of the cell line and drug behavior, and all data being transparently captured in the NFdataportal.org offered the researchers an efficient data-sharing platform.

- *Examples of successful and unsuccessful drug candidates tested on SYNODOS:* SYNODOS has tested a selection of rationally selected drug candidates with mixed results. Some drugs showed promising activity in certain models, while they were less effective in others, highlighting the importance of using multiple models to capture the diversity of NF2-SWN tumors [38]. On the other hand, SYNODOS has identified several promising candidates that have advanced to the Takeda – CTF co-funded platform-basket clinical trial (INTUITT-NF2, NCI, etc.), such as Brigatinib, which was later shown to target the focal adhesion kinase (FAK) pathway in NF2-SWN [39].

- *NCATS drug screening platform and MIPE oncology library screen:* The National Center for Advancing Translational Sciences (NCATS) has been pivotal in accelerating drug discovery through its innovative screening programs. One of its critical assets is the Mechanism Interrogation PlatE (MIPE) library of compounds [40, 41], which includes FDA-approved oncology drugs, and compounds in clinical development and investigational preclinical stage. The compounds in the MIPE collection were annotated for their nominal target, which enables target analysis of hits from each cell line screened. This library facilitates both repurposing drugs for cancers as well as providing valuable pharmacological information on targets and pathways critical for the survival of cancers that are potential therapeutic targets. This library collection is particularly relevant for rare diseases like NF2-SWN, where repurposing existing drugs could significantly shorten the path to effective treatments, and oncology pathways are highly relevant to NF2-SWN. The following steps were involved in the NF2-SWN MIPE library screen:

  - *Cell line selection:* All drugs were screened on NF2-negative schwannoma and meningioma cell lines provided by members of the Synodos NF2.

  - *Drug screening:* The MIPE library, containing over 191 FDA-approved oncology drugs, was systematically tested on the selected cell lines using a cell viability assay in a high-through screening plate format (1536-well per plate). High throughput screening (HTS) in high plate density enables the test of each drug across a range of concentrations to determine its potency and efficacy as cytostatic/cytotoxic drug, for each cell line. This HTS platform allowed rapid identification of compounds that inhibit cell growth or induce cell death in NF2-negative schwannoma and meningioma models.

- *Comprehensive integrated analysis of screening data to increase success rates:* A comprehensive analysis was performed to prioritize active compounds from the dose-response screens. Compounds were first assigned a curve response class using a classifier algorithm developed at NCATS that enables quick bucketing of compounds based on potency and efficacy across the different cell lines [42]. Further analysis of the active compounds based on target enabled pharmacological grouping of the hits from the screen. Finally, high-quality hits from the screens were prioritized based on whether they were approved, clinical, or preclinical development stage. Compiled screening data were discussed by Synodos NF2 group members including, basic research, chemists, biologists, and clinicians, for a final selection of promising inhibitors, which were then taken for further validation, including kinome analysis, investigation target engagement, and pathway regulation *in vitro*, and animal model testing.

5.2.1 *Promising inhibitors identified*

- *Brigatinib:* One of the most surprising and promising hits from the NCATS MIPE screen was Brigatinib, a drug FDA-approved as an ALK (anaplastic lymphoma kinase) inhibitor for lung cancer [43–45]. However, in the context of NF2-SWN, Brigatinib's efficacy was demonstrated to stem from its inhibition of FAK (focal adhesion kinase), a critical enzyme involved in cell signaling, survival, and proliferation in Merlin-deficient cells [18]. Brigatinib's promising preclinical results have led to its inclusion in the INTUITT-NF2 platform-basket trial. This trial confirmed Brigatinib's efficacy in a broader NF2-SWN patient population, mainly in meningioma and non-vestibular schwannoma [39].

- *Other Drug Candidates:* Sapanisertib (TAK-228) and vistusertib (AZD2014) are both mTOR C1/C2 inhibitors that demonstrated significant activity in NF2-SWN models in cell and animal models. Visuterstib even showed clinical efficacy [46]. Despite their promise, both sapanisertib and vistusertib were shelved by their respective companies due to strategic shifts in focus and disappointing clinical trial results in other cancer types. However, their efficacy in NF2-SWN models suggests that these drugs may still have potential if revisited with appropriate dose adjustments and in combination with other therapies. Given the unmet need in NF2-SWN and the mechanistic rationale for targeting mTOR C1/C2 [11, 47], there is significant potential for revisiting sapanisertib and vistusertib. Future studies could explore optimal dosing strategies, combination therapies with FAK inhibitors like Brigatinib, or new formulations that enhance drug delivery to tumors.

- *Future Opportunities:* The findings from the Synodos platform underscore the critical need for a comprehensive, integrated, and efficient preclinical testing platforms that can better predict clinical outcomes for NF2-SWN. This section outlines the future directions for research and collaboration in the field.

6. Establishing an efficient preclinical testing platform

- *Discussion on the future of the CTF preclinical hub:* The Children's Tumor Foundation (CTF) is leading efforts to continuously expand its preclinical hub dedicated to NF (including NF1, NF2-SWN, and non-NF2-SWN). This hub provides a public-private partnership ecosystem for testing drug candidates across various models, including patient-derived xenografts, organoids, and advanced cell lines. CTF offers an accurate, predictive, and standardized testing environment that can efficiently de-risk drug discovery and development for pharmaceutical and biotech companies.

- *How this hub can serve as a global model for other rare diseases:* While the CTF hub is focused on NF, its structure and approach could serve as a model for other rare diseases. The hub can help accelerate drug development in diseases with limited patient populations and high unmet needs by providing access to high-quality preclinical models and standardized testing protocols.

- *Potential collaborations with academic and industry stakeholders:* The success of the CTF preclinical hub relies on strong partnerships with academic institutions, contract research organizations, pharmaceutical/biotech companies, and regulatory agencies. Collaborative efforts are aimed at streamlining the transition from preclinical testing to clinical trials. Establishing these partnerships has shown to be crucial for the hub's success.

- *Development of target product profile:* with the increasing number of preclinically validated drug treatments, there is a need for well-established Target Product Profiles (TPP). The main elements of TPP include each indication/manifestation, drug dosage and administration, clinical outcome, and tolerability. It may also include regulatory and commercial considerations. TPPs set clear optimal, acceptable, and minimal drug property expectations and will assist in making critical decisions during the drug discovery and development process.

- *Incentivizing companies:* Detailed Strategies for Encouraging Pharmaceutical Companies to reposition their shelved assets (https://www.statnews.com/2023/06/27/drug-repurposing-repositioning-rare-diseases/). One of the biggest challenges in rare disease drug development is the reluctance of pharmaceutical companies to reposition shelved assets. Several strategies could be employed to overcome this, including offering financial incentives, such as tax credits or grants, increased Environmental Social Governance (ESG) scores, and regulatory incentives, such as fast-track designations and extended market exclusivity.

- *Potential regulatory and financial incentives:* the orphan drug Designation and the pediatric voucher in the United States and similar legislation in other countries provide a framework for incentivizing drug development in rare diseases. Expanding these programs to include specific incentives for companies repurposing shelved drugs could help bring more treatments to patients with NF2-SWN.

- *Transparent decision-making:* There needs to be more discussion on the Need for Open-Access Data and Collaborative Decision-Making in Rare Disease Research.

DOI: http://dx.doi.org/10.5772/intechopen.1007882

Transparent decision-making and open-access data have been shown to be essential for advancing research in rare diseases like NF2-SWN (www.nfdataportal.org). By making data from preclinical studies, clinical trials, and real-world evidence available to the broader research community, stakeholders can better identify promising therapies and avoid duplication of effort.

Examples of Successful Transparent Decision-Making in Other Fields: The COVID-19 pandemic highlighted the importance of transparency and collaboration in accelerating drug development. Initiatives like the Open Science COVID-19 Data Portal and the ACT Accelerator (https://www.who.int/initiatives/act-accelerator) showcased how sharing data and resources can lead to faster and more effective solutions. Applying these principles to rare disease research could similarly expedite progress toward rare disease treatments.

7. Conclusion

In conclusion, the Synodos preclinical screening platform and the INTUITT-NF2 platform-basket trial have laid a strong foundation for future drug development efforts in NF2-SWN. By establishing a robust preclinical testing platform, incentivizing pharmaceutical companies to release shelved assets, and promoting transparent decision-making, the field is poised to make significant strides toward finding effective treatments for this challenging disease.

Acknowledgements

The authors want to acknowledge the Synodos NF2 Consortium: Robert Allaway, Steve P. Angus, Roberta L. Beauchamp, Marga Bott, Sarah S. Burns, Annemarie Carlstedt, Long-Sheng Chang, Xin Chen, Patrick A. Desouza, Serkan Erdin, Cristina Fernandez-Valle, Justin Guinney, Stephen J. Haggarty, Gary L. Johnson, Salvatore La Rosa, Helen Morrison, Marco Nievo, Alejandra M. Petrilli, Abhishek Pratap, Vijaya Ramesh, Noah Sciaky, Anat Stemmer-Rachamimov, Tim J. Stuhlmiller, Michael E. Talkowski, D. Bradley Welling, Charles W. Yates, Jon S. Zawistowski, Wen-Ning Zhao, Xiaohu Zhang, and Craig Thomas.

Conflict of interest

The authors declare no conflicts of interest.

Author details

Annette Bakker[1]*, D. Wade Clapp[2], James Gusella[3], Jaishri Blakeley[4], Scott Plotkin[5] and Marc Ferrer[6]

1 Children's Tumor Foundation, NY, USA

2 Indiana University School of Medicine, Indianapolis, IN, USA

3 Harvard Medical School, Boston, MA, USA

4 Johns Hopkins University School of Medicine, Baltimore, MD, USA

5 Harvard Medical School, Mass General Research Institute, Boston, MA, USA

6 National Center for Advancing Translational Sciences, Rockville, MD, USA

*Address all correspondence to: abakker@ctf.org

References

[1] Forde C, Smith MJ, Burghel GJ, Bowers N, Roberts N, Lavin T, et al. *NF2*-related schwannomatosis and other schwannomatosis: An updated genetic and epidemiological study. Journal of Medical Genetics. 2024;**61**(9):856-860. DOI: 10.1136/jmg-2024-110065

[2] Plotkin SR, Messiaen L, Legius E, Pancza P, Avery RA, Blakeley JO, et al. Updated diagnostic criteria and nomenclature for neurofibromatosis type 2 and schwannomatosis: An international consensus recommendation. Genetics in Medicine. 2022;**24**(9):1967-1977. DOI: 10.1016/j.gim.2022.05.007

[3] Agnihotri S, Jalali S, Wilson MR, Danesh A, Li M, Klironomos G, et al. The genomic landscape of schwannoma. Nature Genetics. 2016;**48**(11):1339-1348. DOI: 10.1038/ng.3688

[4] Parry DM, MacCollin MM, Kaiser-KupferMI, PulaskiK, NicholsonHS, Bolesta M, et al. Germ-line mutations in the neurofibromatosis 2 gene: Correlations with disease severity and retinal abnormalities. American Journal of Human Genetics. 1996;**59**(3):529-539

[5] Vlashi R, Sun F, Zheng C, Zhang X, Liu J, Chen G. The molecular biology of NF2/Merlin on tumorigenesis and development. The FASEB Journal. 2024;**38**(13):e23809. DOI: 10.1096/fj.202400019RR

[6] Wu M, Hu L, He L, Yuan L, Yang L, Zhao B, et al. The tumor suppressor NF2 modulates TEAD4 stability and activity in hippo signaling via direct interaction. The Journal of Biological Chemistry. 2024;**300**(5):107212. DOI: 10.1016/j.jbc.2024.107212

[7] Bassiri K, Ferluga S, Sharma V, Syed N, Adams CL, Lasonder E, et al. Global proteome and Phospho-proteome analysis of Merlin-deficient meningioma and Schwannoma identifies PDLIM2 as a novel therapeutic target. eBioMedicine. 2017;**16**:76-86. DOI: 10.1016/j.ebiom.2017.01.020

[8] Zhao F, Li SW, Zhang S, Li P, Zhao C, Zhao XB, et al. Phase II trial of icotinib in adult patients with neurofibromatosis type 2 and progressive vestibular schwannoma. Journal of Neurosurgery. 2022;**138**(6):1680-1687. DOI: 10.3171/2022.9.JNS22699

[9] Curto M, Cole BK, Lallemand D, Liu CH, McClatchey AI. Contact-dependent inhibition of EGFR signaling by Nf2/Merlin. The Journal of Cell Biology. 2007;**177**(5):893-903. DOI: 10.1083/jcb.200703010

[10] James MF, Han S, Polizzano C, Plotkin SR, Manning BD, Stemmer-Rachamimov AO, et al. NF2/merlin is a novel negative regulator of mTOR complex 1, and activation of mTORC1 is associated with meningioma and schwannoma growth. Molecular and Cellular Biology. 2009;**29**(15):4250-4261. DOI: 10.1128/MCB.01581-08

[11] Sagers JE, Beauchamp RL, Zhang Y, Vasilijic S, Wu L, DeSouza P, et al. Combination therapy with mTOR kinase inhibitor and dasatinib as a novel therapeutic strategy for vestibular schwannoma. Scientific Reports. 2020;**10**(1):4211. DOI: 10.1038/s41598-020-60156-6

[12] Huegel J, Dinh CT, Martinelli M, Bracho O, Rosario R, Hardin H, et al. CUDC907, a dual phosphoinositide-3 kinase/histone deacetylase inhibitor, promotes apoptosis of NF2 Schwannoma cells. Oncotarget. 2022;**13**:890-904. DOI: 10.18632/oncotarget.28254

[13] Yang H, Hall SRR, Sun B, Zhao L, Gao Y, Schmid RA, et al. NF2 and canonical hippo-YAP pathway define distinct tumor subsets characterized by different immune deficiency and treatment implications in human pleural mesothelioma. Cancers (Basel). 2021;**13**(7):1561. DOI: 10.3390/cancers13071561

[14] Laraba L, Hillson L, de Guibert JG, Hewitt A, Jaques MR, Tang TT, et al. Inhibition of YAP/TAZ-driven TEAD activity prevents growth of NF2-null schwannoma and meningioma. Brain. 2023;**146**(4):1697-1713. DOI: 10.1093/brain/awac342

[15] Burns SS, Akhmametyeva EM, Oblinger JL, Bush ML, Huang J, Senner V, et al. Histone deacetylase inhibitor AR-42 differentially affects cell-cycle transit in meningeal and meningioma cells, potently inhibiting NF2-deficient meningioma growth. Cancer Research. 2013;**73**(2):792-803. DOI: 10.1158/0008-5472.CAN-12-1888

[16] Welling DB, Collier KA, Burns SS, Oblinger JL, Shu E, Miles-Markley BA, et al. Early phase clinical studies of AR-42, a histone deacetylase inhibitor, for neurofibromatosis type 2-associated vestibular schwannomas and meningiomas. Laryngoscope Investigative Otolaryngology. 2021;**6**(5):1008-1019. DOI: 10.1002/lio2.643

[17] Morris KA, Golding JF, Axon PR, Afridi S, Blesing C, Ferner RE, et al. Bevacizumab in neurofibromatosis type 2 (NF2) related vestibular schwannomas: A nationally coordinated approach to delivery and prospective evaluation. Neurooncology Practice. 2016;**3**(4):281-289. DOI: 10.1093/nop/npv065

[18] Chang LS, Oblinger JL, Smith AE, Ferrer M, Angus SP, Hawley E, et al. Brigatinib causes tumor shrinkage in both NF2-deficient meningioma and schwannoma through inhibition of multiple tyrosine kinases but not ALK. PLoS One. 2021;**16**(7):e0252048. DOI: 10.1371/journal.pone.0252048

[19] Vittoria MA, Shenk EM, O'Rourke KP, Bolgioni AF, Lim S, Kacprzak V, et al. A genome-wide microRNA screen identifies regulators of tetraploid cell proliferation. Molecular Biology of the Cell. 2018;**29**(13):1682-1692. DOI: 10.1091/mbc.E18-02-0141

[20] Cioffi JA, Yue WY, Mendolia-Loffredo S, Hansen KR, Wackym PA, Hansen MR. MicroRNA-21 overexpression contributes to vestibular schwannoma cell proliferation and survival. Otology & Neurotology. 2010;**31**(9):1455-1462. DOI: 10.1097/MAO.0b013e3181f20655

[21] Hannan CJ, Lewis D, O'Leary C, Donofrio CA, Evans DG, Roncaroli F, et al. The inflammatory microenvironment in vestibular schwannoma. Neuro-oncology Advances. 2020;**2**(1):vdaa023. DOI: 10.1093/noajnl/vdaa023

[22] Plotkin SR, Blakeley JO, Dombi E, Fisher MJ, Hanemann CO, Walsh KS, et al. Achieving consensus for clinical trials: The REiNS international collaboration. Neurology. 2013;**81**(21 Suppl. 1):S1-S5. DOI: 10.1212/01.wnl.0000435743.49414.b6

[23] Gross AM, Plotkin SR, Widemann BC. REiNS international collaboration. Neurofibromatosis clinical trials-REiNS collaboration 2020 recommendations: Looking Back and moving ahead. Neurology. 2021;**97**(7 Suppl. 1):S1-S3. DOI: 10.1212/WNL.0000000000012429

[24] Dilwali S, Patel PB, Roberts DS, Basinsky GM, Harris GJ, Emerick KS,

et al. Primary culture of human Schwann and schwannoma cells: Improved and simplified protocol. Hearing Research. 2014;**315**:25-33. DOI: 10.1016/j.heares.2014.05.006

[25] van de Weijer LL, Ercolano E, Zhang T, Shah M, Banton MC, Na J, et al. A novel patient-derived meningioma spheroid model as a tool to study and treat epithelial-to-mesenchymal transition (EMT) in meningiomas. Acta Neuropathologica Communications. 2023;**11**(1):198. DOI: 10.1186/s40478-023-01677-9

[26] Giovannini M, Robanus-Maandag E, van der Valk M, Niwa-Kawakita M, Abramowski V, Goutebroze L, et al. Conditional biallelic Nf2 mutation in the mouse promotes manifestations of human neurofibromatosis type 2. Genes & Development. 2000;**14**(13):1617-1630

[27] Gehlhausen JR, Park SJ, Hickox AE, Shew M, Staser K, Rhodes SD, et al. A murine model of neurofibromatosis type 2 that accurately phenocopies human schwannoma formation. Human Molecular Genetics. 2015;**24**(1):1-8. DOI: 10.1093/hmg/ddu414

[28] Saydam O, Ozdener GB, Senol O, Mizrak A, Prabhakar S, Stemmer-Rachamimov AO, et al. A novel imaging-compatible sciatic nerve schwannoma model. Journal of Neuroscience Methods. 2011;**195**(1):75-77. DOI: 10.1016/j.jneumeth.2010.10.021

[29] Püttmann S, Senner V, Braune S, Hillmann B, Exeler R, Rickert CH, et al. Establishment of a benign meningioma cell line by hTERT-mediated immortalization. Laboratory Investigation. 2005;**85**(9):1163-1171. DOI: 10.1038/labinvest.3700307

[30] Lazaro O, Li S, Carter W, Awosika O, Robertson S, Hickey BE, et al. A novel induced pluripotent stem cell model of Schwann cell differentiation reveals *NF2*-related gene regulatory networks of the extracellular matrix. bioRxiv [Preprint]. 2024. DOI: 10.1101/2024.05.02.591952

[31] López Vásquez CE, Gray C, Henry C, Munro MJ. Modelling meningioma using organoids: A review of methodologies and applications. The Organ. 2023;**2**:218-230. DOI: 10.3390/organoids2040017

[32] Neufeld L, Yeini E, Reisman N, Shtilerman Y, Ben-Shushan D, Pozzi S, et al. Microengineered perfusable 3D-bioprinted glioblastoma model for in vivo mimicry of tumor microenvironment. Science Advances. 2021;**7**(34):eabi9119. DOI: 10.1126/sciadv.abi9119

[33] Tung YT, Chen YC, Derr K, Wilson K, Song MJ, Ferrer M. A 3D bioprinted human neurovascular unit model of glioblastoma tumor growth. Advanced Healthcare Materials. 2024;**13**(15):e2302831. DOI: 10.1002/adhm.202302831

[34] Xie Z, Chen M, Lian J, Wang H, Ma J. Glioblastoma-on-a-chip construction and therapeutic applications. Frontiers in Oncology. 2023;**13**:1183059. DOI: 10.3389/fonc.2023.1183059

[35] Giovannini M, Bonne N-X, Vitte J, Chareyre F, Tanaka K, et al. mTORC1 inhibition delays growth of neurofibromatosis type 2 schwannoma. Neuro-Oncology. 2014;**16**(4):493-504. DOI: 10.1093/neuonc/not242

[36] Karajannis MA, Legault G, Hagiwara M, Giancotti FG, Filatov A, Derman A, et al. Phase II study of everolimus in children and adults with neurofibromatosis type 2 and progressive vestibular schwannomas. Neuro-Oncology. 2014;**16**(2):292-297. DOI: 10.1093/neuonc/not150

[37] Bakker A, Browder V, Jarvis K, La Rosa S, Nievo M. Collaboration in research for rare disease: How nonprofits can be the changemakers. British Journal of Cancer Research. 2022;**5**(1):540-549. DOI: 10.31488/bjcr.174

[38] Synodos for NF2 Consortium, Allaway R, Angus SP, Beauchamp RL, Blakeley JO, Bott M, et al. Traditional and systems biology based drug discovery for the rare tumor syndrome neurofibromatosis type 2. PLoS One. 2018;**13**(6):e0197350. DOI: 10.1371/journal.pone.0197350

[39] Plotkin SR, Yohay KH, Nghiemphu PL, Dinh CT, Babovic-Vuksanovic D, Merker VL, et al. Brigatinib in *NF2*-related Schwannomatosis with progressive Tumors. The New England Journal of Medicine. 2024;**390**(24):2284-2294. DOI: 10.1056/NEJMoa2400985

[40] Mathews Griner LA, Guha R, Shinn P, Young RM, Keller JM, Liu D, et al. High-throughput combinatorial screening identifies drugs that cooperate with ibrutinib to kill activated B-cell-like diffuse large B-cell lymphoma cells. Proceedings of the National Academy of Sciences of the United States of America. 2014;**111**(6):2349-2354. DOI: 10.1073/pnas.1311846111

[41] Ferrer M, Gosline SJC, Stathis M, Zhang X, Guo X, Guha R, et al. Pharmacological and genomic profiling of neurofibromatosis type 1 plexiform neurofibroma-derived schwann cells. Scientific Data. 2018;**5**:180106. DOI: 10.1038/sdata.2018.106

[42] Inglese J, Auld DS, Jadhav A, Johnson RL, Simeonov A, Yasgar A, et al. Quantitative high-throughput screening: A titration-based approach that efficiently identifies biological activities in large chemical libraries. Proceedings of the National Academy of Sciences of the United States of America. 2006;**103**(31):11473-11478. DOI: 10.1073/pnas.0604348103

[43] Spencer SA, Riley AC, Matthew A, Di Pasqua AJ. Brigatinib: Novel ALK inhibitor for non-small-cell lung cancer. The Annals of Pharmacotherapy. 2019;**53**(6):621-626

[44] Gupta N, Hanley MJ, Griffin RJ, Zhang P, Venkatakrishnan K, Sinha V. Clinical pharmacology of Brigatinib: A next-generation anaplastic lymphoma kinase inhibitor. Clinical Pharmacokinetics. 2023;**62**(8):1063-1079

[45] Bronte G, Cafaro A, Pasini L, et al. Brigatinib in the first-line treatment of ALK+ metastatic NSCLC: Safety and efficacy. Expert Review of Anticancer Therapy. 2021;**21**(8):809-817

[46] Jordan JT, Orr CC, Thalheimer RD, Cambillo JV, Beauchamp RL, Shaikh G, et al. Prospective phase II trial of the dual mTORC1/2 inhibitor vistusertib for progressive or symptomatic meningiomas in persons with neurofibromatosis 2. Neuro-oncology Advances. 2023;**5**(1):vdad041. DOI: 10.1093/noajnl/vdad041

[47] Bhattacharyya S, Oblinger JL, Beauchamp RL, Kosa L, Robert F, Plotkin SR, et al. Preclinical evaluation of the third-generation, bi-steric mechanistic target of rapamycin complex 1-selective inhibitor RMC-6272 in *NF2*-deficient models. Neuro-oncology Advances. 2024;**6**(1):vdae024. DOI: 10.1093/noajnl/vdae024

Chapter 8

Design Strategies for Smart Hydrogels: From Concept to Application

Bharti Sapra, Shama Parveen, Ashok Kumar Tiwari and Om Silakari

Abstract

Smart hydrogels are extensively used in the medical field due to their flexible behavior with respect to external stimuli. This chapter includes advancements in smart hydrogels for biomedical applications and computational approaches that can be used to prepare smart hydrogel. Numerous polymers, having the ability to form a cross-linking network structure, swell and retain the water when exposed to a physiological environment, are used to manufacture the hydrogels. However, hydrogels exhibit numerous benefits but have various drawbacks such as low tensile strength, limited drug loading capacity, limited long-term stability, limited mechanical strength. Hence, to overcome these limitations, researchers have the opinion to redesign the hydrogel into stimuli-responsive hydrogel (smart hydrogel), having significant characteristics with respect to the external environment such as pH, temperature, light. Researchers use various techniques and design strategies such as polymerization techniques and cross-linking techniques for the production of hydrogels. Some in silico approaches such as molecular dynamic (MD) simulation, computational chemistry simulation, bioinformatics and biomolecular modeling, polymer simulation package, have been recently explored by various researchers in order to optimize this delivery system. These tools can expedite the process of selection and production of smart hydrogels for various biomedical applications.

Keywords: smart hydrogel, external stimuli, computational techniques, stimuli responsive, bioinformatics, biomolecular modeling

1. Introduction

Nowadays, hydrogels are commonly used as a targeted drug delivery vehicle due to its potential applications in the fields of medicine, tissue engineering, wound healing, biosensors, inflammation relief, soft robotic components, etc. Basically, hydrogels are networks of hydrophilic polymeric chains having significant potential of swelling when exposed to a physiological environment and capable of retaining large amounts of water within its cross-linked structure. Because of the large volume of water retained within its structure, it shows the property of flexibility which imitates the natural tissue of the body [1, 2].

The hydrogels have numerous benefits such as the release of drugs at a controlled rate, biodegradability, nontoxic nature, and significant biocompatibility and hydrophilicity [3]. The physical and structural integrity of hydrogels is mainly due to the property of chemical cross-linkage and physical interactions within the molecular structure of the hydrogel network [4]. Despite its various benefits, they have certain limitations in the field of drug delivery which are described in **Figure 1**.

These limitations can be overcome by redesigning the hydrogels into smart hydrogels for more efficient targeted drug delivery. The development of smart biomaterials has attained great attention in recent years because of their increased applications in the field of personalized medications for improved treatment regimes [5, 6].

Stimuli-responsive hydrogels are composed of smart polymers that have the ability to change their physical and mechanical properties in their network structure when exposed to stimuli such as pH, temperature, light, electric field, magnetic field, and biological stimuli (enzyme, antigens, DNA, etc.) and initiate the release of drug [2, 7]. Hydrogels are flexible in the route of administration, have the ability to protect the drug from the environment, are highly biocompatible, and have the ability to protect the drug from the environment [8].

In order to formulate smart hydrogels recently, the *in-silico* studies have been performed for optimal designing. Some key aspects of *in-silico* studies such as molecular dynamics (MD) simulations have been explored for investigating the interaction between particular atoms and hydrogels network [9], for predicting the equilibrium swelling ratio, rate of swelling, and how all these properties can be altered under different circumstances. Diffusion simulations are another way to study the solute diffusion inside the hydrogel network [10]. Dug release modeling (computational modeling) can be used to simulate the drug release from stimuli-responsive hydrogels in order to predict the release kinetics, drug distribution within the hydrogel network [11]. To understand the biocompatibility and bioactivity of hydrogel materials in the areas of tissue engineering and regenerative medicines simulations that investigate the interaction between hydrogels and biological components such as proteins, tissues and cells are required [12].

Alinejad and researchers had formulated a system for doxorubicin (DOX) through smart polymers coated grapheme (G) having the ability to control the release of drug

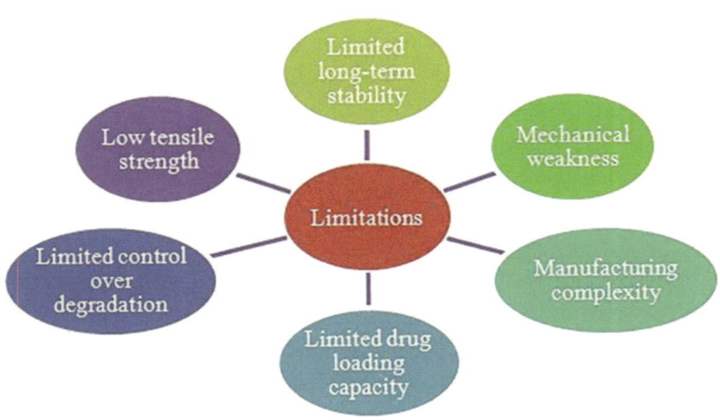

Figure 1.
Limitations of hydrogel.

and water-soluble characteristics. The molecular dynamics (MD) simulations and density functional theory (DFT) calculations have been used to predict the significant combination between G-DOX and polyethyleneimine. After completion of the study, results showed that the binding energy of DOX on graphene in the presence of polyethyleneimine (PPEI) significantly increased by about 20% when exposed to neutral conditions, while in the acidic environment, the drug absorption became weaker and immediately removed from the system and G-DOX complex could come in contact with cancer cells [12].

2. Types of smart hydrogels

There are numerous types of smart hydrogels e.g., on the basis origin of polymers (natural, synthetic, or mixture of both), cross-linking techniques (physical cross-linking, chemical cross-linking, hybrid i.e., chemical/physical cross-linking), methods of preparation (irradiation method, free radical method, solution casting method, interpenetrating method) and stimuli responsive behavior (biochemical stimuli hydrogels, physically stimuli hydrogels, chemically stimuli hydrogels), etc. [7, 13]. **Figure 2** depicts the types of smart hydrogels. **Table 1** summarizes a few examples of delivery systems that are representatives of smart hydrogels.

Aycan and Almedar developed chitosan-based pH-responsive hydrogel for controlled release of amoxicillin which had been modified with bone ash. These hydrogels were fabricated by the process of photopolymerization and are composed of poly (ethylene glycol) diacrylate (PEGDA) and chitosan-grafted-glycidyl methacrylate (CTS-g-GMA) under the exposure of UV light. Amoxycillin was used as the model drug in this study. After evaluating the parameters of the resulting formulation, it was elucidated that the hydrogels exhibited improved mechanical characteristics and therefore, performed as a novel drug carrier for treating gastric ulcers [32].

Hu and co-researchers developed ion-responsive, Ca^{2+}-based superabsorbent hydrogels as the cementing material for better compressive strength and self-healing properties. The swelling behavior was found to be inversely related to the concentration of calcium as the concentration of calcium increased from 0.014 to 0.2 mol/L the swelling was found to decrease from 15 to 5 g/g. However, an increase in the concentration of calcium decreased the compressive strength of the cement material from 28.49 MPa to 17.8% MPa due to air more entrapment. The study further revealed that Ca-Alg released

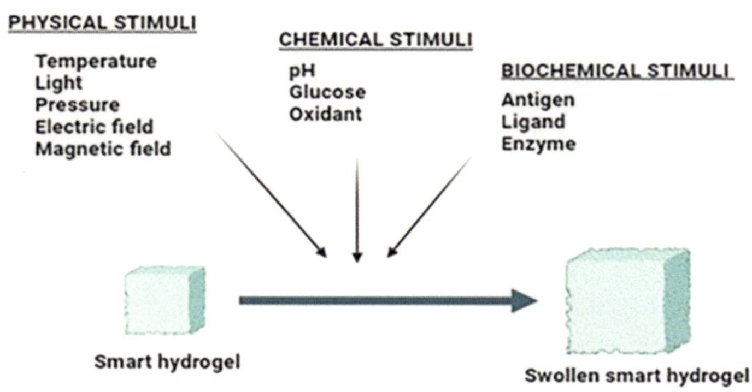

Figure 2.
Representation of swelling of smart hydrogels under the external stimuli.

Type	Examples	Key points	Merits	Demerits	Applications	Reference
Temperature responsive	Pluronic, Poloxamer, Glycero-phosphate, PEG, PAA	Due to the Change in temperature, the equilibrium between a hydrophilic and hydrophobic portion of the cross-linked chain is disturbed and the rate of sol-gel transformation is increased	Controlled degradation, easy functionalization, unique physical properties similar to external matrix	Thermolabile drugs are not good candidates, compatibility problems, poor mechanical strength	Tissue engineering, Intraocular lenses, In biotechnology for protein purification	[14, 15]
pH-responsive	Guar gum, chitosan, succinate, PDEAEMA, PMAA, PVA, kappa-carrageenan	Existence of high electrostatic repulsion among polymeric chains and alteration in their hydrophobicity is the major factor responsible for pH dependent swelling/deswelling behavior	Sustained release of drugs, biocompatible, Improved stability, hydrophilicity, suitable for thermolabile drugs	Low mechanical strength, susceptibility to toxicity, alteration in swelling ratio	Wound and skin healing, inflammation responsive, drug delivery, sensing	[16–18]
Magnetic-field responsive	Magnetic nanoparticle, Xanthan bovine serum, albumin magnetic nanoparticles	Magnetic nanoparticles are made up of magnetite, maghemite, and ferrite	Controlled release of drugs	Complexity of control, limited mechanical strength, biocompatibility concern, temperature sensitivity	Tissue engineering, microfluidics, drug delivery	[19, 20]
Light responsive	Azo benzene bovine albumin, triphenylmethane leuco derivatives	Initiating the sol-gel transformation due to external stimuli of either UV or visible	Biocompatible, minimize invasive procedure	Limited long-term stability, limited structural integrity, Poor mechanical strength, chances of chromophore leakage that are noncovalently bound	Optical delivery, self-sterilization and self-cleaning	[21–23]

Type	Examples	Key points	Merits	Demerits	Applications	Reference
Biochemical responsive	Phenyl borate derivative, insulin, poly(2-hydroxyethylmethacrylate-co-N,N-dimethacrylate) in combination with glucose oxidase	Alteration in the pH and concentration of biomolecules exhibit the potential of expanding polyelectrolytes which are responsible for the swelling or deswelling properties	Controlled release, high specificity, high affinity, biocompatibility	Restricted to stimuli specificity, Biocompatible limited loading capacity	In the Insulin delivery system, cell culture, tissue engineering, sensing, drug delivery	[24–26]
Electric field responsive	Agarose, chondroitin sulfate, carbomer, calcium alginate, xanthan gum, hyaluronic acid	Bending or deswelling based upon structure and arrangement of hydrogel with respect to electrode in the presence of electric field	Controlled release, biocompatibility, minimal invasiveness	Susceptible to tissue damage, electrode dependency, biocompatibility problems, low mechanical strength	In drug delivery, and cosmetics as thickener and stabilizer, in buccal drug delivery, as emulsion stabilizer in suspension and creams	[27–29]
Ion-responsive	Polyacrylamide, sodium alginate, Ag^+, Cu^{2+}, Co^{2+}, Ca^{2+}, carboxymethylcellulose	Ion concentration within the hydrogel altered along with variation in ionic strength, swelling and deswelling takes place which is responsible for the release of drug	Biocompatibility, responsiveness to multiple environmental stimuli, high specificity in sensing and responding	Limited mechanical strength, low extend of stability, highly susceptible to cause cytotoxicity, manufacturing process very complex	As a carrier for targeted delivery of drugs, used as bioadhesives and hemostats, actuation and robotics, in regeneration of tissues and bones	[30, 31]

PEG = Polyethylene glycol, PAA = Poly(acrylic acid), PDEAEMA = Poly(2-(diethylamino)ethyl methacrylate, PMAA = Poly(methacrylic acid), PVA = polyvinyl alcohol.

Table 1.
Types of smart hydrogels.

the Ca^{2+} ions to facilitate the precipitation capacity of calcium silicate hydrates, which was responsible for a more efficient healing process [33].

3. Techniques for preparation of smart hydrogels

The researchers have worked hard to produce smart hydrogels by changing their physicochemical characteristics as they respond to various physical, chemical, and biological stimuli [34]. The hydrophilic polymeric network has to be cross-linked in some way to create the hydrogel having an elastic structure. Therefore, hydrogels can be produced by any technique (e.g., copolymerization/cross-linking free radical polymerization) that generates the cross-linked polymer. Generating the main chain free radical in the presence of ionizing radiation that may be rejoined together in order to produce cross-linked junctions and electrostatic interaction, crystallite formation or entanglements and all of these are physical processes to produce cross-linked polymeric structure [35, 36].

3.1 Polymerization techniques

In polymerization, monomers are chemically combined to create a large cross-linked chain or network of molecules i.e., polymer. The manufacturing of hydrogels could be obtained either through a single-step polymerization process that simultaneously involves the cross-linking along with polymerization of monomers having polyfunctional characteristics or through multistep process that involves the aggregation of polymers having the ability to react and cross-linking either independently or by reaction using appropriate cross-linkers [37].

3.1.1 Chain growth polymerization technique

Chemically cross-linked hydrogels are manufactured by the process of chain growth polymerization through the mechanism of free radicals. Three stages of the polymerization process that are used for the preparation of hydrogel are initiation, propagation, and termination. In the process of free radical polymerization, the monomers having hydrophilic double-bond carbon are involved [38]. The free radical polymerization techniques used to prepare hydrogels are:

3.1.1.1 Bulk polymerization

Due to its simple mechanism, bulk polymerization is commonly used for the preparation of hydrogels. In this technique, the liquid monomers and monomer-soluble initiators undergo polymerization along with a small number of cross-linkers. Radiation, ultraviolet light, and/or chemical catalysts, act as the initiators for the polymerization process. The conversion rate of the bulk polymerization process can be regulated through an appropriate concentration of initiators. The strategy to control the conversion rate of bulk polymerization is to interrupt the polymerization reaction. However, it is not suitable for large-scale production. Therefore, suspension, solution, emulsion techniques of the polymerization process can be extensively used for the manufacturing of hydrogels. **Figure 3** enumerates various techniques used for preparation of hydrogels.

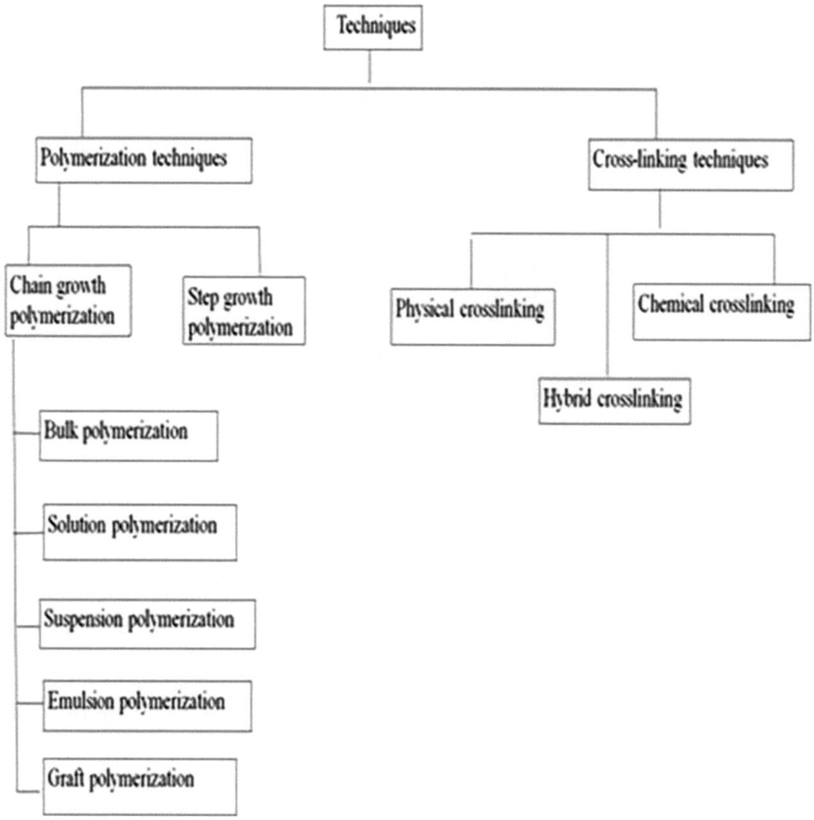

Figure 3.
Descriptive representation of various techniques for preparation of hydrogels.

There are various polymerization techniques such as solution polymerization, suspension polymerization, and grafting polymerization that have been used in the preparation of smart hydrogels from a cross-linked network of synthetic polymers such as polylactic acid, polyvinyl pyrrolidone (PVP), polyethylene oxide (PEO), polyacrylic acid, or some natural polymers such as carrageenan, pectin, hyaluronic acid, Alginic acid and chondroitin sulfate [39]. A common method of preparation of hydrogels is described in **Figure 4**.

3.1.1.2 Solution polymerization

To manufacture hydrogel, in the process of solution polymerization, the monomer (ionic or neutral in nature) along with solvent (such as water-ethanol mixture, water, and benzyl alcohol) and cross-linkers are combined together [38].

3.1.1.3 Suspension polymerization

In the suspension polymerization technique, the droplets are produced in the range of 0.1–5 mm diameter by constantly stirring of solution containing low hydrophilic-lipophilic equilibrium and monomers that are insoluble in order to

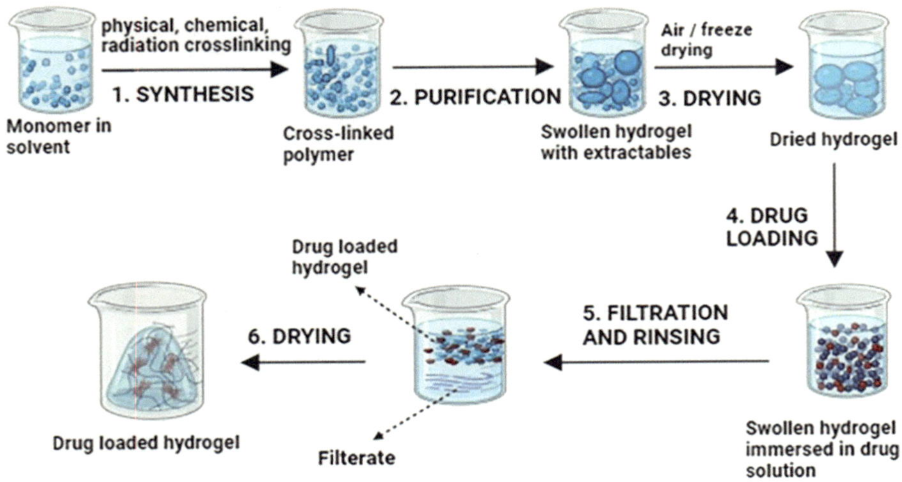

Figure 4.
Representation of the method of preparation of hydrogels.

prepare hydrogels. The carboxymethyl cellulose (CMC), polyvinyl alcohol (PVA), and methylcellulose (MC) are the colloidal agents having protective in nature, and are used to prevent the coalescence of droplets in the process of suspension polymerization. This technique also known as 'inverse-suspension polymerization technique is most commonly used for the preparation of hydrogels [40].

3.1.1.4 Emulsion polymerization

In this technique, the initiators (water-soluble), cross-linkers, surfactants, and monomers (slightly soluble in water and entirely hydrophobic in nature) are involved in manufacturing the hydrogel [41]. A droplet size of 0.1–3 μm can be obtained by this technique which is smaller than the droplets that are produced from the process of suspension polymerization [34].

3.1.1.5 Graft polymerization

Bulk polymerization produces the hydrogel having poor mechanical characteristics. So, the graft polymerization technique is used to significantly increase the mechanical characteristics of the hydrogel by surface-coated hydrogel onto the stronger support. This technique produces free radicals on a more enduring support surface, monomers undergo the polymerization process instantaneously and lead to the formation of a monomer chain which is attached to the support surface by a covalent bond. Numerous kinds of polymeric support can be used to produce hydrogels through graft polymerization [42].

3.1.2 Step growth polymerization technique

In this technique, the monomers that have various functional groups which might create the links *via* covalent bonds can initiate the single-step polymerization process that can be used in the production of hydrogels. Due to the homogenous and

Polymerization technique	Types	Benefits	Drawbacks	Reference
Chain growth polymerization	Bulk polymerization	High degree of polymerization and rate of conversion	Costly, limited mechanical characteristics	[1, 43, 44]
	Solution polymerization	Carried out at room temperature, heat transfer can be controlled in a better way, synthesizing the superabsorbent hydrogel composed of cellulose, solvent acts as a heat sinker.	Sophisticated technique, mono/poly- disparity due to uncontrolled hydrolytic and thermal cleavage	[34, 38, 45]
	Suspension polymerization	A more frequently used technique; microspheres (droplets) or powder are obtained through this technique due to lack of grinding.	Thermodynamically unstable, suspending agents are required	[2, 46, 47]
	Emulsion polymerization	Significant heat transfer, rate of reaction can be easily controlled, high product purity	Limited solvent compatibility, high energy consumption	[48–50]
	Graft polymerization	Enhance the mechanical properties, improve the adhesion of polymers	Required high energy radicals to initiate the reaction which leads to chain scission, challenges on scale-up production	[51–53]
Step-growth polymerization		High thermal stability, lower level of residual monomers, accommodate vide range of polymers	Slow rate of reaction, limited control over molecular weight distribution	[54–56]

Table 2.
Summary of different polymeric techniques used for hydrogel production.

cooperative features of the polymeric network, the light-degradable hydrogels having significant mechanical properties such as ductileness, shear strain, integrity, and tensile strength are prepared through the process of step-growth polymerization [38].

Table 2 summarizes different research investigations involving different techniques for hydrogel formation.

3.2 Cross-linking techniques

In cross-linking, two or more molecules combine chemically through a covalent bond in order to create a 3D network structure. Cross-linking techniques are widely used to manufacture smart hydrogels because these techniques prevent the hydrophilic portion of hydrogels from disintegrating in an aqueous medium that is necessary to

Type	Benefits	Drawbacks	Reference
Physical cross-linking	Non-destructive due to the absence of chemical reaction, cost-effective, biocompatible, easily fabricated, potential for *in situ* formulation	Limited mechanical strength, dependency on specific stimuli, and limited cross-linking density control. Slower response time as compared to chemical cross-linking	[57–59]
Chemical cross-linking	High mechanical strength, long-term stability, long-lasting response, prevents undesirable reaction due to substrate specificity	Difficulty in achieving homogeneity, high susceptibility of toxicity, challenge to precisely controlling the kinetics of stimulus responsiveness, Difficulty in terminating the reaction, Extreme reaction time	[59–61]
Hybrid cross-linking	Enhanced swelling/deswelling kinetics reduced toxicity, high compatibility with biologically active components, versatile to stimuli-responsive	Patent and intellectual property issue because of high reaction time, and complexity in designing and optimizing the hydrogels because of the hybrid cross-linking of polymers	[62–64]

Table 3.
Descriptive representation of benefits and drawbacks of cross-linking techniques.

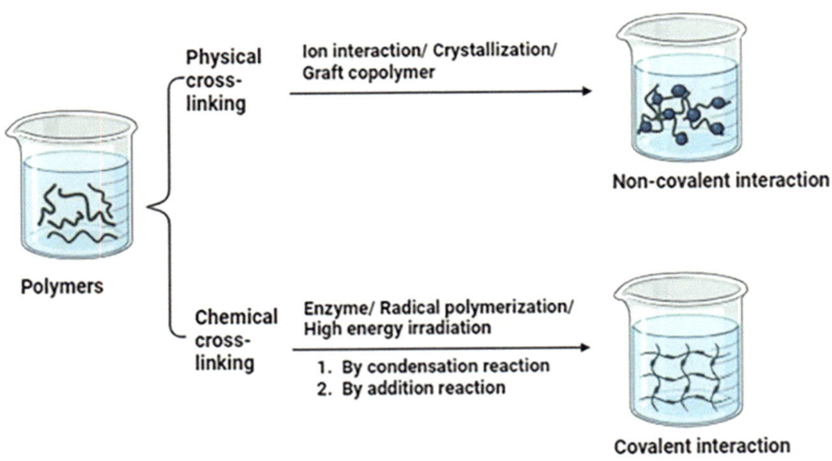

Figure 5.
Mechanism of cross-linking techniques for preparation of hydrogels.

manufacture the hydrogel with high mechanical properties. **Table 3** explains the advantages and limitations of cross-linking techniques [65]. Different types of cross-linking techniques depending upon the mechanism of cross-linking are described in **Figure 5**.

4. *In-silico* approaches for synthesis of stimuli-responsive hydrogels

Applying the computational technique to design and optimize the molecular structure and composition of materials of hydrogels is an integral part of *in-silico* approaches for designing stimuli-responsive hydrogels [66]. Before manufacturing the hydrogels in laboratories, these approaches may help the researchers to estimate the physicochemical characteristics and functionality of hydrogels. There are numerous *in-silico* techniques as well as tools that can be used to create the stimuli-responsive hydrogels.

4.1 Molecular dynamics (MD) simulation

In recent years, molecular dynamics simulations have proved to be significant in molecular biology and the development of drugs. The movement of every atom within a protein or other biomolecular system over time can be predicted by molecular dynamics simulation on the basis of interatomic interactions [67]. CHARMM, AMBER, NAMD, and GROMACS are simulation tools that are most extensively used to predict the conformational changes in bimolecular process, ligand binding, location of atoms in biomolecules, and protein folding [68].

Rezaeisada and co-investigators have performed MD simulations to find out the interaction between curcumin and nano-micelle made up of PNIPAAm-b-PEG copolymers in order to create the smart drug delivery system. Drug entrapment efficiency, interatomic interactions, and behavior of polymers with curcumin in an aqueous medium were investigated by using the GROMACS software. After conducting the study, the results showed that the phase change temperature for PNIPAAm-b-PEG was found to be in the range of 300–305 k, whereas with 9% polymer and at 310 k the optimum diameter of developed micelles is equivalent to 4.36 nm. The solubility of the drug increased by 88% in the presence of polymer [69].

4.2 Computational chemistry simulation

In computational chemistry simulation, helps or assists in finding or screening the functional monomers that have appropriate composition, structure, and reference

Simulation technique	Software tool	Applications	References
Molecular dynamics (|MD) Simulations	GROMACS	Simulation of the motion of molecules in hydrogels	[10, 12, 71]
	LAMMPS	Open source MD simulator for modeling complex hydrogel systems	[9, 72, 73]
	NAMD	Simulation programs designed for high-performance molecular dynamics	[72, 74, 75]
Monte Carlo Simulations	CHARMM	Include Monte Carlo simulations for studying hydrogel systems	[72, 76]
	ABF-MC (Adaptive Biasing Force Monte Carlo)	Specifically designed in order to study the free energy landscapes of complex systems	[60, 75]
Finite Element Analysis (FEA)	COMSOL metaphysics	Used to model the mechanical behavior of hydrogels and their response to external stimuli	[77, 78]
	ANSYS	Extensively used for quantum calculations and for prediction of molecular characteristics of hydrogels (polymer network, cross-linking swelling behavior, and stimuli-responsive moieties)	[25, 79]

Simulation technique	Software tool	Applications	References
Polymer simulation packages	ESPReeSo	Specialized software in order to simulate the complex fluids and polymers	[80, 81]
	Phyton	Software having multipurpose programming language that is used in polymer simulation by writing the custom analysis script	[36, 82]
	Material studio	Software for polymer simulation, used to study the behavior and characteristics of polymers	[83, 84]
Bioinformatics and biomolecular modeling	AutoDock Vina	Used in molecular docking studies in order to predict how molecules interact with hydrogel network	[66, 85, 86]
Computational chemistry simulations	GAMESS or Gaussian	To calculate the electronic and structural properties of individual monomers and polymers for hydrogel production	[87, 88]
Density Functional Theory (DFT)	NanoDCAL and RESCU	DFT calculations provide the electronic structure, bonding, and reactivity of components that are used in hydrogel production	[12]

Table 4.
Summary of various in-silico simulation techniques along with software tools and applications.

compounds by using computer-like research tools [70]. There are many computational simulation software that can be used to serve this purpose are summarized in **Table 4**.

4.3 Monte Carlo simulations

Monte Carlo simulation is a group of computer-determined stochastic sampling-based techniques that can be used to approximate the difficulties that arise in mathematical concepts and modeling for statistical purposes [89].

4.4 Polymer simulations packages

Computer-based programs are used by scientists in order to find out the distinctive features and molecular behavior of polymer material. There are various tools that are included in this simulation package such as Material Studio, ESPReeSo, phyton, etc.

The choice of software depends on the complexity of hydrogel systems, materials used for production of stimuli-responsive hydrogels, and the aim of specific research. Researchers may also use these tools in combination in order to gain a significant understanding of the stimuli responsive behavior of hydrogels.

5. Simulation tools

Simulation tools are software programs or computational models that are used to simulate biological, chemical, or physical processes in a computer-based environment. These tools enable researchers to predict the behavior of complex systems without the need for costly and time-consuming experimentation. Some commonly used

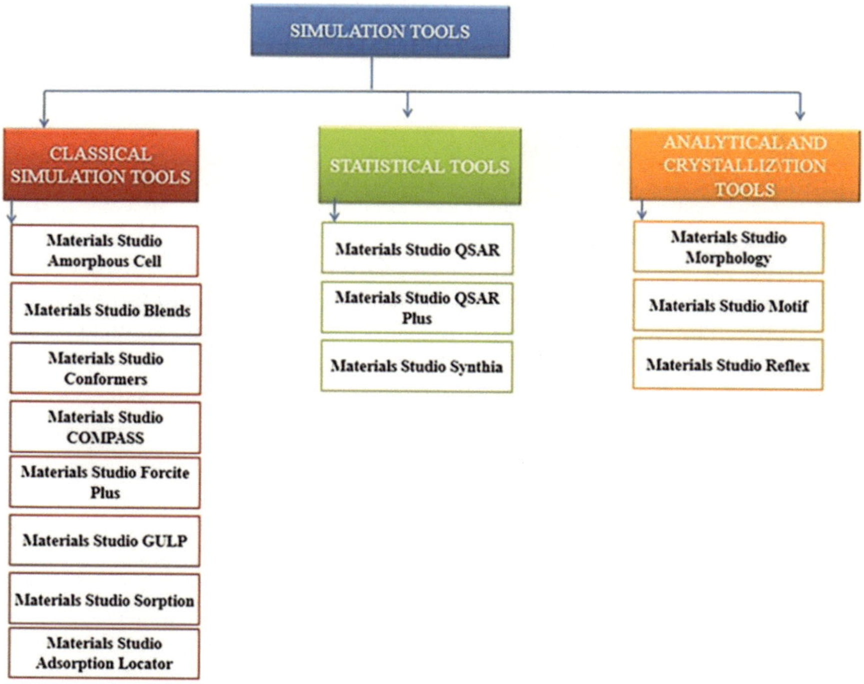

Figure 6.
Types of simulation tools.

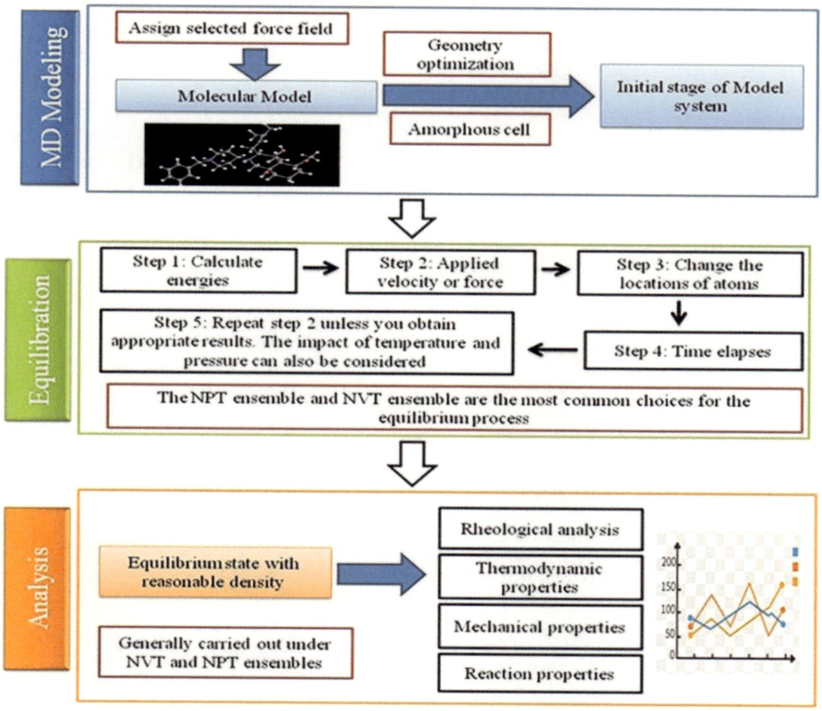

Figure 7.
Brief representation of procedure for MD simulation of materials.

in silico simulation tools across various fields are described in **Figure 6** [90]. **Figure 7** is a brief representation of the procedure used for the MD simulation of materials.

6. Applications of stimuli responsive hydrogels

Smart stimuli-responsive hydrogel polymers have distinctive features such as biocompatibility, hydrophilicity, swelling/deswelling character, and biodegradability which contribute to their ability to be used for different kinds of biomedical applications which include tissue engineering, biosensors, actuators and targeted drug delivery [91, 92]. The hydrogels that acquire self-healing, high mechanical strength, and high flexibility can be manufactured by surface functionalization, by adding the functional material and modifying the functional group. **Table 5** describes the biomedical applications of different polymers [79].

Class of smart hydrogel	Smart hydrogel polymers	Application area	References
Temperature responsive	• Poly(N-isopropylacrylamide) (PNIPAAm), • Methylacrylate gelatin (GelMA), • Polyacrylamide (PAAM) • Poly(N-isopropylacrylamide) (PNIPAAm) • Poly(N-isopropylacrylamide) (PNIPAAm)-Hydrophobically • Associated polyacrylamide (HAPAM) hydrogel (HAPAM-PNIPAAM)	Microfluidic actuators, Skin wound healing, Targeted drug delivery Biosensors for smart compression	[93, 94]
Coumarin-loaded Light responsive hydrogel	• Polyacrylamide (PAAM) • Poly(N,N-dimethylacrylamide (PDMA) • Poly(N-isopropylacrylamide) (PNIPAAM)	Controlled and targeted delivery of drugs for the treatment of cancer, Engineering of neural tissue, For numerous biomedical applications	[95, 96]
Electric responsive hydrogels	• Poly(3,4-ethylenedioxythiophene) (PEDOT) conductive • polymer layer, • Carboxymethyl chitosan (CMCH) • Chitosan (CH)	Biosensors, targeted drug delivery, tissue engineering, used in cosmetics to release skincare responsive formulation, used in wound healing	[97–100]
Magnetic responsive hydrogels	• N-isopropylacrylamide (NIPAAM) • Methylacrylate gelatin (GelMA) • Polyacrylamide (PAAM) • Polyethylene glycol (PEG)	3D printing, micro actuators, Used for delivery of biomolecules, food supplements, cosmetics products, controlled release of drugs, as a container for catalyst	[101–103]

Class of smart hydrogel	Smart hydrogel polymers	Application area	References
Ultrasound responsive hydrogels	• Poly(acrylamidoglycolic acid) (PAGA) • Polyethylene Glycol (PEG)	Used in cancer therapy, Used in *in-vitro* cell culture, used as a coating on implants and medical devices	[104, 105]
Strain/pressure responsive hydrogels	• Carboxy Meyhylcellulose (CMC), • Polyacrylamide (PAAM) • Poly(acrylamide-co-Lauryl Methacrylate) (P(AAM-co-LMA))	Used in strain sensors and wearable biosensors	[106, 107]
Glucose-responsive hydrogels	• Poly(N-vinylpyrrolidone-co-dimethylamino)ethyl acrylate-co-3-(acrylamido)PBA • Phenylboronic acid-grafted γ-Polyglutamic acid (PBA-PGA)	For targeted delivery of 3D cells, proteins, and biocompatible substances, served as glucose-sensitive components in diagnostic assays and sensors	[108–110]
Enzyme responsive hydrogels	• -Polypeptides (PLys-b-(PHIS-co-PBLG)-PLys-b-(PHIS-co-PBLG)-b-Plys) • Chitosan (CH) • Hyaluronic Acid (HA) • Gelatin	Used in tissue engineering, tumor microenvironment, and in 3D cell culture	[111, 112]
Antigens/antibody-responsive hydrogels	• Polyacrylamide (PAAM) • N-(9-fluorenylmethoxycarbonyl) • L, L –diphenylalanine (Fmoc-FF)	As sensing elements in biosensors, applied in tissue engineering and regenerative medicines, used for antibody immobilization	[113–115]
pH-responsive hydrogels	• Poly(acrylamidoglycolic acid) (PAGA) • Poly(acrylamidoglycolic acid) (PAGA) • pre-gel hydrogel solution 80 mol% acrylamide, 8 mol% 3-acrylamidophenylboronic acid, 10 mol% N-[3-(dimethylamino)propyl] methacrylamide, 2 mol% N, N0-Methylenebisacrylamide	Used in tissue cartilage engineering, used in detecting devices for environmental pollutants and disease indicators in drinking water	[116–119]
Ionic strength and redox-responsive hydrogels	• Ethylene glycol dimethacrylate (EGDMA) • Polyethylene Glycol (PEG) • Chitosan (CH) • Gelatin	Used in diagnostic assay, targeted drug delivery, biosensors, tissue engineering, and regenerative medicines. In cell sorting and isolation	[111, 120, 121]

Table 5.
Summary of recently developed smart hydrogels employed for biomedical applications.

Smart hydrogels are a major breakthrough in biomedical use because they can react to outside influences, providing better functionality compared to conventional hydrogels. Smart hydrogels have been developed to react to different external triggers like pH, temperature, light, ionic strength, electric fields, and magnetic fields [122]. These responsive hydrogels can experience reversible chemical or physical alterations, enabling precise drug release, focused therapy and improved tissue engineering uses. For instance, hydrogels sensitive to temperature can release drugs based on the body's temperature changes, ensuring a steady and controlled release pattern [42]. Hydrogels composed of polymers like poly(N-isopropylacrylamide) (PNIPAM), chitosan, and hyaluronic acid can mimic the properties of biological membranes, acting as scaffolds for cell growth and tissue regeneration. These polymers form cross-linked network structures that swell and retain water when exposed to physiological conditions, creating a supportive environment for cells. However, traditional hydrogels face limitations such as low tensile strength, limited drug loading capacity, and restricted long-term stability [123]. In order to optimize the hydrogel with respect to stimuli, *in silico* tools and software have been used. Material studio software has been using to select suitable polymers in different ratios for the preparation of smart hydrogels with desirable mechanical characteristics [124].

Recently many reviews have been compiled to comprehend the significance of hydrogels in tissue engineering, biomedical applications, ocular drug delivery systems, and also in biomimetic formulations. Recent reports have shown that hydrogel wound dressings might be an effective strategy for treating diabetic wounds due to their excellent hydrophilicity, good drug loading ability, and sustained drug release properties. Due to the intricacy of diabetic wounds, antibiotics, and other medications are frequently combined with hydrogel dressings in clinical practice, although the hostile environment easily hinders these medications [125]. Smart biological hydrogels show great promise as topical drug delivery systems for oral mucosal lesions, offering sustained drug release, increased therapeutic efficacy, and minimized systemic complications. The potential benefits of biological polymer-based hydrogels make them an exciting area of research for oral mucosal lesion treatment as well as for ocular delivery [126, 127].

7. Conclusion

Due to high bioavailability, response to specific stimuli and resemblance to actual body tissues, smart/stimuli-responsive hydrogels have demonstrated considerable promise in medicinal areas, biomedical applications especially in the delivery of drugs at the target site, and tissue engineering [2]. Stimuli-responsive hydrogels have the ability to deliver hydrophilic as well as hydrophobic drugs regulate the kinetics of drug release and significantly protect the drugs that are sensitive to specific conditions [128].

Production of stimuli responsive hydrogel for innovative drug delivery systems is challenging and requires expertise from the different kinds of production areas [129]. Recently researchers have started using *in silico* tools for rational designing of hydrogel by predicting and optimizing their performance and physicochemical characteristics [10].

8. Future perspective

In the area of smart hydrogel, *in silico* software might play a potential role in the rational design of smart hydrogel. Enhanced machine learning algorithms can predict the properties and behavior of new polymers more accurately, allowing for faster and more efficient screening of potential candidates. In addition, polymer designs can be optimized for specific applications e.g., for improving drug loading capacity, release profiles, and biocompatibility. Future research would definitely focus on integrating multi-scale modeling, from the molecular level to the macroscopic level, to provide a more comprehensive understanding of polymer behavior in biological systems. *In silico* tools can be used to design tailor-made polymer according to individual patient's needs, considering factors like genetics, disease state, and personal preferences. *In silico* tools can also predict the biocompatibility of new polymers, reducing the need for extensive *in vivo* testing and accelerating the development of safe materials.

Conflicts of interest

The authors declare that they have no conflict of interest.

Statement of Human and Animal Rights (including Statement of Informed Consent).

This article does not contain any studies with human and animal subjects performed by any of the authors.

Author details

Bharti Sapra*, Shama Parveen, Ashok Kumar Tiwari and Om Silakari
Department of Pharmaceutical Science's and Drug Research, Punjabi University, Patiala, Punjab, India

*Address all correspondence to: bhartijatin2000@yahoo.co.in

References

[1] Ahmed EM. Hydrogel: Preparation, characterization, and applications: A review. Journal of Advanced Research. 2015;**6**(2):105-121

[2] Bordbar-Khiabani A, Gasik M. Smart hydrogels for advanced drug delivery systems. International Journal of Molecular Sciences. 2022;**23**(7):3665

[3] Ghasemiyeh P, Mohammadi-Samani S. Hydrogels as drug delivery systems; pros and cons. Trends in Pharmaceutical Sciences. 2019;**5**(1):7-24

[4] Jacob S, Nair AB, Shah J, Sreeharsha N, Gupta S, Shinu P. Emerging role of hydrogels in drug delivery systems, tissue engineering and wound management. Pharmaceutics. 2021;**13**(3):357

[5] Khan F, Tanaka M. Designing smart biomaterials for tissue engineering. International Journal of Molecular Sciences. 2017;**19**(1):17

[6] Montoya C, Du Y, Gianforcaro AL, Orrego S, Yang M, Lelkes PI. On the road to smart biomaterials for bone research: Definitions, concepts, advances, and outlook. Bone Research. 2021;**9**(1):12

[7] Ullah F, Othman MB, Javed F, Ahmad Z, Akil HM. Classification, processing and application of hydrogels: A review. Materials Science and Engineering: C. 2015;**57**:414-433

[8] Sood N, Bhardwaj A, Mehta S, Mehta A. Stimuli-responsive hydrogels in drug delivery and tissue engineering. Drug Delivery. 2016;**23**(3):748-770

[9] Rukmani SJ, Anstine DM, Munasinghe A, Colina CM. An insight into structural and mechanical properties of idealnetworked poly (ethylene glycol)–peptide hydrogels from molecular dynamics simulations. Macromolecular Chemistry and Physics. 2020;**221**(3):1900326

[10] Bina A, Raissi H, Hashemzadeh H, Farzad F. Conjugation of a smart polymer to doxorubicin through a pH-responsive bond for targeted drug delivery and improving drug loading on graphene oxide. RSC Advances. 2021;**11**(31):18809-18817

[11] Fu IW, Markegard CB, Nguyen HD. Solvent effects on kinetic mechanisms of self-assembly by peptide amphiphiles via molecular dynamics simulations. Langmuir. 2015;**31**(1):315-324

[12] Alinejad A, Raissi H, Hashemzadeh H. Development and evaluation of a pH-responsive and water-soluble drug delivery system based on smart polymer coating of graphene nanosheets: An in silico study. RSC Advances. 2020;**10**(52):31106-31114

[13] Bashir S, Hina M, Iqbal J, Rajpar AH, Mujtaba MA, Alghamdi NA, et al. Fundamental concepts of hydrogels: Synthesis, properties, and their applications. Polymers. 2020;**12**(11):2702

[14] Fang JY, Chen JP, Leu YL, Hu JW. Temperature-sensitive hydrogels composed of chitosan and hyaluronic acid as injectable carriers for drug delivery. European Journal of Pharmaceutics and Biopharmaceutics. 2008;**68**(3):626-636

[15] Bolla PK, Rodriguez VA, Kalhapure RS, Kolli CS, Andrews S, Renukuntla J. A review on pH and temperature responsive gels and other less explored drug delivery systems.

Journal of Drug Delivery Science and Technology. 2018;**46**:416-435

[16] Rizwan M, Yahya R, Hassan A, Yar M, Azzahari AD, Selvanathan V, et al. pH sensitive hydrogels in drug delivery: Brief history, properties, swelling, and release mechanism, material selection and applications. Polymers. 2017;**9**(4):137

[17] Liang Y, Zhao X, Ma PX, Guo B, Du Y, Han X. pH-responsive injectable hydrogels with mucosal adhesiveness based on chitosan-grafted-dihydrocaffeic acid and oxidized pullulan for localized drug delivery. Journal of Colloid and Interface Science. 2019;**536**:224-234

[18] Han Z, Wang P, Mao G, Yin T, Zhong D, Yiming B, et al. Dual pH-responsive hydrogel actuator for lipophilic drug delivery. ACS Applied Materials & Interfaces. 2020;**12**(10):12010-12017

[19] Sun Z, Song C, Wang C, Hu Y, Wu J. Hydrogel-based controlled drug delivery for cancer treatment: A review. Molecular Pharmaceutics. 2019;**17**(2):373-391

[20] Li Z, Li Y, Chen C, Cheng Y. Magnetic-responsive hydrogels: From strategic design to biomedical applications. Journal of Controlled Release. 2021;**335**:541-556

[21] Giammanco GE, Sosnofsky CT, Ostrowski AD. Light-responsive iron (III)–polysaccharide coordination hydrogels for controlled delivery. ACS Applied Materials & Interfaces. 2015;7(5):3068-3076

[22] Lv SW, Liu Y, Xie M, Wang J, Yan XW, Li Z, et al. Near-infrared light-responsive hydrogel for specific recognition and photothermal site-release of circulating tumor cells. ACS Nano. 2016;**10**(6):6201-6210

[23] Roth-Konforti ME, Comune M, Halperin-Sternfeld M, Grigoriants I, Shabat D, Adler-Abramovich L. UV light–responsive peptide-based supramolecular hydrogel for controlled drug delivery. Macromolecular Rapid Communications. 2018;**39**(24):1800588

[24] Debele TA, Mekuria SL, Tsai HC. Polysaccharide based nanogels in the drug delivery system: Application as the carrier of pharmaceutical agents. Materials Science and Engineering: C. 2016;**68**:964-981

[25] Wang D, Hu Y, Liu P, Luo D. Bioresponsive DNA hydrogels: Beyond the conventional stimuli responsiveness. Accounts of Chemical Research. 2017;**50**(4):733-739

[26] Bajpai AK, Kankane S, Chouhan R, Goswami S. Biological stimulus-responsive hydrogels. In: Polymeric Biomaterials. USA: CRC Press; 2020. pp. 1187-1214

[27] Li Y, Sun Y, Xiao Y, Gao G, Liu S, Zhang J, et al. Electric field actuation of tough electroactive hydrogels cross-linked by functional triblock copolymer micelles. ACS Applied Materials & Interfaces. 2016;**8**(39):26326-26331

[28] Xue B, Qin M, Wang T, Wu J, Luo D, Jiang Q, et al. Electrically controllable actuators based on supramolecular peptide hydrogels. Advanced Functional Materials. 2016;**26**(48):9053-9062

[29] Zhu QL, Dai CF, Wagner D, Daab M, Hong W, Breu J, et al. Distributed electric field induces orientations of nanosheets to prepare hydrogels with elaborate ordered structures and programmed deformations. Advanced Materials. 2020;**32**(47):2005567

[30] Soppimath KS, Aminabhavi TM, Dave AM, Kumbar SG, Rudzinski WE. Stimulus-responsive "smart" hydrogels as novel drug delivery systems. Drug Development and Industrial Pharmacy. 2002;**28**(8):957-974

[31] Li Z, Zhou Y, Li T, Zhang J, Tian H. Stimuli-responsive hydrogels: Fabrication and biomedical applications. Viewpoints. 2022;**3**(2):20200112

[32] Aycan D, Alemdar N. Development of pH-responsive chitosan-based hydrogel modified with bone ash for controlled release of amoxicillin. Carbohydrate Polymers. 2018;**184**:401-407

[33] Hu M, Guo J, Du J, Liu Z, Li P, Ren X, et al. Development of Ca2+–based, ion-responsive superabsorbent hydrogel for cement applications: Self-healing and compressive strength. Journal of Colloid and Interface Science. 2019;**538**:397-403

[34] El-Husseiny HM, Mady EA, Hamabe L, Abugomaa A, Shimada K, Yoshida T, et al. Smart/stimuli-responsive hydrogels: Cutting-edge platforms for tissue engineering and other biomedical applications. Materials Today Bio. 2022;**13**:100186

[35] Singh SK, Dhyani A, Juyal D. Hydrogel: Preparation, characterization and applications. The Pharma Innovations. 2017;**6**(6, Part A):25

[36] Sahu N, Gupta D, Nautiyal U. Hydrogel: Preparation, characterization and applications. Asian Pacific Journal of Nursing and Health Sciences. 2020;**3**(1):1-1

[37] Hennink WE, van Nostrum CF. Novel crosslinking methods to design hydrogels. Advanced Drug Delivery Reviews. 2012;**64**:223-236

[38] Ranganathan N, Bensingh RJ, Kader MA, Nayak SK. Synthesis and properties of hydrogels prepared by various polymerization reaction systems. In: Polymers and Polymeric Composites: A Reference Series. Springer; 2018. pp. 1-25

[39] Zhao L, Xiao C, Gai G, Ding J. Glucose-sensitive polymer nanoparticles for self-regulated drug delivery. Chemical Communications. 2016;**52**(49):7633-7652

[40] Liu J, Jiang L, He S, Zhang J, Shao W. Recent progress in PNIPAM-based multi-responsive actuators: A mini-review. Chemical Engineering Journal. 2022;**433**:133496

[41] Young RJ, Lovell PA. Introduction to Polymers. Boca Raton, United States: CRC Press; 2011

[42] Sikdar P, Uddin MM, Dip TM, Islam S, Hoque MS, Dhar AK, et al. Recent advances in the synthesis of smart hydrogels. Materials Advances. 2021;**2**(14):4532-4573

[43] Achilias DS, Verros GD. Modeling of diffusion-controlled reactions in free radical solution and bulk polymerization: Model validation by DSC experiments. Journal of Applied Polymer Science. 2010;**116**(3):1842-1856

[44] Carraher CE Jr. Carraher's Polymer Chemistry. Boca Raton, United States: CRC Press; 2017

[45] Chanda M. Introduction to Polymer Science and Chemistry: A Problem-Solving Approach. Boca Raton, United States: CRC Press; 2006

[46] Liu M, Liang R, Zhan F, Liu Z, Niu A. Preparation of superabsorbent slowrelease nitrogen fertilizer by inverse suspension polymerization. Polymer International. 2007;**56**(6):729-737

[47] Akhtar MF, Hanif M, Ranjha NM. Methods of synthesis of hydrogels... A review. Saudi Pharmaceutical Journal. 2016;**24**(5):554-559

[48] Watanabe T, Song C, Murata K, Kureha T, Suzuki D. Seeded emulsion polymerization of styrene in the presence of water-swollen hydrogel microspheres. Langmuir. 2018;**34**(29):8571-8580

[49] Zhong JX, Clegg JR, Ander EW, Peppas NA. Tunable poly (methacrylic acid-co-acrylamide) nanoparticles through inverse emulsion polymerization. Journal of Biomedical Materials Research Part A. 2018;**106**(6):1677-1686

[50] Hu X, Karnetzke J, Fassbender M, Drücker S, Bettermann S, Schroeter B, et al. Smart reactors–combining stimuli-responsive hydrogels and 3D printing. Chemical Engineering Journal. 2020;**387**:123413

[51] Nasef MM, Gürsel SA, Karabelli D, Güven O. Radiation-grafted materials for energy conversion and energy storage applications. Progress in Polymer Science. 2016;**63**:1-41

[52] Wohlhauser S, Delepierre G, Labet M, Morandi G, Thielemans W, Weder C, et al. Grafting polymers from cellulose nanocrystals: Synthesis, properties, and applications. Macromolecules. 2018;**51**(16):6157-6189

[53] Messina MS, Messina KM, Bhattacharya A, Montgomery HR, Maynard HD. Preparation of biomolecule-polymer conjugates by grafting-from using ATRP, RAFT, or ROMP. Progress in Polymer Science. 2020;**100**:101186

[54] Lu C, Wang C, Yu J, Wang J, Chu F. Two-step 3D-printing approach toward sustainable, repairable, fluorescent shape-memory thermosets derived from cellulose and rosin. ChemSusChem. 2020;**13**(5):893-902

[55] Rizwan M, Gilani SR, Durani AI, Naseem S. Materials diversity of hydrogel: Synthesis, polymerization process and soil conditioning properties in agricultural field. Journal of Advanced Research. 2021;**33**:15-40

[56] Gao Y, Peng K, Mitragotri S. Covalently crosslinked hydrogels via step-growth reactions: Crosslinking chemistries, polymers, and clinical impact. Advanced Materials. 2021;**33**(25):2006362

[57] Li X, Zhang Y, Yang Q, Li D, Zhang G, Long S. Agar/PAAc-Fe 3+ hydrogels with pH-sensitivity and high toughness using dual physical cross-linking. Iranian Polymer Journal. 2018;**27**:829-840

[58] Bustamante-Torres M, Romero-Fierro D, Arcentales-Vera B, Palomino K, Magaña H, Bucio E. Hydrogels classification according to the physical or chemical interactions and as stimuli-sensitive materials. Gels. 2021;**7**(4):182

[59] Xue X, Hu Y, Wang S, Chen X, Jiang Y, Su J. Fabrication of physical and chemical crosslinked hydrogels for bone tissue engineering. Bioactive Materials. 2022;**12**:327-339

[60] Wang J, Chen M, Zhao H, Zhang H, Yang X. Stimuli-responsive supramolecular gels based on the self-assembly of stigmasterol-ferrocene derivative. Colloid and Interface Science Communications. 2020;**39**:100321

[61] Ghorpade VS. Preparation of hydrogels based on natural polymers via chemical reaction and cross-linking. In:

Hydrogels Based on Natural Polymers. Netherlands: Elsevier; 2020. pp. 91-118

[62] Yu Y, Feng R, Li J, Wang Y, Song Y, Tan G, et al. A hybrid genipin-crosslinked dual-sensitive hydrogel/nanostructured lipid carrier ocular drug delivery platform. Asian Journal of Pharmaceutical Sciences. 2019;**14**(4):423-434

[63] Zhang F, Hu C, Kong Q, Luo R, Wang Y. Peptide–/drug-directed self-assembly of hybrid polyurethane hydrogels for wound healing. ACS Applied Materials & Interfaces. 2019;**11**(40):37147-37155

[64] Vasile C, Pamfil D, Stoleru E, Baican M. New developments in medical applications of hybrid hydrogels containing natural polymers. Molecules. 2020;**25**(7):1539

[65] El-Sherbiny IM, Khalil IA, Ali IH. Updates on stimuli-responsive polymers: Synthesis approaches and features. In: Polymer Gels: Science and Fundamentals. Springernature; 2018. pp. 129-146

[66] Pereira A, Valdés-Muñoz E, Marican A, Cabrera-Barjas G, Vijayakumar S, Valdés O, et al. Rational design of hydrogels for cationic antimicrobial peptide delivery: A molecular modeling approach. Pharmaceutics. 2023;**15**(2):474

[67] Hollingsworth SA, Dror RO. Molecular dynamics simulation for all. Neuron. 2018;**99**(6):1129-1143

[68] Hospital A, Goñi JR, Orozco M, Gelpí JL. Molecular dynamics simulations: Advances and applications. Advances and Applications in Bioinformatics and Chemistry. 2015;**8**:37-47

[69] Rezaeisadat M, Bordbar AK, Omidyan R. Molecular dynamics simulation study of curcumin interaction with nano-micelle of PNIPAAm-b-PEG co-polymer as a smart efficient drug delivery system. Journal of Molecular Liquids. 2021;**332**:115862

[70] Marć M, Kupka T, Wieczorek PP, Namieśnik J. Computational modeling of molecularly imprinted polymers as a green approach to the development of novel analytical sorbents. TrAC Trends in Analytical Chemistry. 2018;**98**:64-78

[71] Pronk S, Páll S, Schulz R, Larsson P, Bjelkmar P, Apostolov R, et al. GROMACS 4.5: A high-throughput and highly parallel open source molecular simulation toolkit. Bioinformatics. 2013;**29**(7):845-854

[72] Ribeiro D, Yuto G, Titotto SL. Analysis about the behavior and modeling of PH-sensitive hydrogels with different ratios of chitosan and polyvinylpyrrolidone. Journal of Materials Science and Chemical Engineering. 2019;**7**(8):64-76

[73] Palkar V, Choudhury CK, Kuksenok O. Development of dissipative particle dynamics framework for modeling hydrogels with degradable bonds. MRS Advances. 2020;**5**(17):927-934

[74] Sedghiniya S, Soleimannejad J, Foroutan M, Ebrahimi M, Naeini VF. AV (iii)-induced metallogel with solvent stimuli-responsive properties: Structural proof-of-concept with MD simulations. RSC Advances. 2021;**11**(58):36801-36813

[75] Shahi S, Roghani-Mamaqani H, Hoogenboom R, Talebi S, Mardani H. Stimuli-responsive covalent adaptable hydrogels based on homolytic bond dissociation and chain transfer reactions. Chemistry of Materials. 2022;**34**(2):468-498

[76] Tsai CC, Payne GF, Shen J. Exploring pH-responsive, switchable crosslinking mechanisms for programming reconfigurable hydrogels based on aminopolysaccharides. Chemistry of Materials. 2018;**30**(23):8597-8605

[77] Morales D, Bharti B, Dickey MD, Velev OD. Bending of responsive hydrogel sheets guided by field-assembled microparticle endoskeleton structures. Small. 2016;**12**(17):2283-2290

[78] Patel H, Chen J, Hu Y, Erturk A. Photo-responsive hydrogel-based re-programmable metamaterials. Scientific Reports. 2022;**12**(1):13033

[79] Deng K, Rohn M, Gerlach G. Design, simulation and characterization of hydrogel-based thermal actuators. Sensors and Actuators B: Chemical. 2016;**236**:900-908

[80] Minina ES, Sánchez PA, Likos CN, Kantorovich SS. The influence of the magnetic filler concentration on the properties of a microgel particle: Zero-field case. Journal of Magnetism and Magnetic Materials. 2018;**459**:226-230

[81] Mantha S, Pillai S, Khayambashi P, Upadhyay A, Zhang Y, Tao O, et al. Smart hydrogels in tissue engineering and regenerative medicine. Materials. 2019;**12**(20):3323

[82] Fortunato ME, Colina CM. Pysimm: A python package for simulation of molecular systems. SoftwareX. 2017;**6**:7-12

[83] Ma Q, Zhang M, Xu X, Meng K, Yao C, Zhao Y, et al. Multiresponsive supramolecular luminescent hydrogels based on a nucleoside/lanthanide complex. ACS Applied Materials & Interfaces. 2019;**11**(50):47404-47412

[84] Wang J, Zhang X, Wang A, Hu X, Deng L, Lou L, et al. The synthesis and simulations of solvent-responsive bilayer hydrogel. Polymer. 2020;**204**:122801

[85] Mallawarachchi S, Gejji V, Sierra LS, Wang H, Fernando S. Electrical field reversibly modulates enzyme kinetics of hexokinase entrapped in an electro-responsive hydrogel. ACS Applied Bio Materials. 2019;**2**(12):5676-5686

[86] Rizvi AS, Murtaza G, Yan D, Irfan M, Xue M, Meng ZH, et al. Development of molecularly imprinted 2D photonic crystal hydrogel sensor for detection of L-Kynurenine in human serum. Talanta. 2020;**208**:120403

[87] Huang W, Tarakanova A, Dinjaski N, Wang Q, Xia X, Chen Y, et al. Design of multistimuli responsive hydrogels using integrated modeling and genetically engineered silk–elastin-like proteins. Advanced Functional Materials. 2016;**26**(23):4113-4123

[88] Yang Z, Yang X, Long R, Li J. Stimulation modulates adhesion and mechanics of hydrogel adhesives. Langmuir. 2021;**37**(23):7097-7106

[89] Chalmers RP, Adkins MC. Writing effective and reliable Monte Carlo simulations with the SimDesign package. The Quantitative Methods for Psychology. 2020;**16**(4):248-280

[90] Sharma S, Kumar P, Chandra R. Applications of BIOVIA materials studio, LAMMPS, and GROMACS in various fields of science and engineering. In: Molecular Dynamics Simulation of Nanocomposites Using BIOVIA Materials Studio, Lammps and Gromacs. Elsevier; 2019. pp. 329-341

[91] Zhu Y, Yao Z, Liu Y, Zhang W, Geng L, Ni T. Incorporation of

ROS-responsive substance P-loaded zeolite imidazolate framework-8 nanoparticles into a Ca2+–cross-linked alginate/pectin hydrogel for wound dressing applications. International Journal of Nanomedicine. 2020;**15**:333-346

[92] Deng X, Korogiannaki M, Rastegari B, Zhang J, Chen M, Fu Q, et al. "Click" chemistry-tethered hyaluronic acid-based contact lens coatings improve lens wettability and lower protein adsorption. ACS Applied Materials & Interfaces. 2016;**8**(34):22064-22073

[93] D'eramo L, Chollet B, Leman M, Martwong E, Li M, Geisler H, et al. Microfluidic actuators based on temperature-responsive hydrogels. Microsystems & Nanoengineering. 2018;**4**(1):1-7

[94] Zhang Y, Chen K, Li Y, Lan J, Yan B, Shi L, et al. High-strength, self-healable, temperature-sensitive, MXene-containing composite hydrogel as a smart compression sensor. ACS Applied Materials & Interfaces. 2019;**11**(50):47350-47357

[95] Kabb CP, O'Bryan CS, Deng CC, Angelini TE, Sumerlin BS. Photoreversible covalent hydrogels for soft-matter additive manufacturing. ACS Applied Materials & Interfaces. 2018;**10**(19):16793-16801

[96] Dong M, Shi B, Liu D, Liu JH, Zhao D, Yu ZH, et al. Conductive hydrogel for a photothermal-responsive stretchable artificial nerve and coalescing with a damaged peripheral nerve. ACS Nano. 2020;**14**(12):16565-16575

[97] Peng L, Liu Y, Huang J, Li J, Gong J, Ma J. Microfluidic fabrication of highly stretchable and fast electro-responsive graphene oxide/polyacrylamide/alginate hydrogel fibers. European Polymer Journal. 2018;**103**:335-341

[98] Xu C, Guan S, Wang S, Gong W, Liu T, Ma X, et al. Biodegradable and electroconductive poly (3, 4-ethylenedioxythiophene)/carboxymethyl chitosan hydrogels for neural tissue engineering. Materials Science and Engineering: C. 2018;**84**:32-43

[99] Gan D, Han L, Wang M, Xing W, Xu T, Zhang H, et al. Conductive and tough hydrogels based on biopolymer molecular templates for controlling in situ formation of polypyrrole nanorods. ACS Applied Materials & Interfaces. 2018;**10**(42):36218-36228

[100] Jiang H, Fan L, Yan S, Li F, Li H, Tang J. Tough and electro-responsive hydrogel actuators with bidirectional bending behavior. Nanoscale. 2019;**11**(5):2231-2237

[101] Liu H, Wang C, Gao Q, Liu X, Tong Z. Magnetic hydrogels with supracolloidal structures prepared by suspension polymerization stabilized by Fe2O3 nanoparticles. Acta Biomaterialia. 2010;**6**(1):275-281

[102] Augurio A, Cortelletti P, Tognato R, Rios A, Levato R, Malda J, et al. A multifunctional nanocomposite hydrogel for endoscopic tracking and manipulation. Advanced Intelligent Systems. 2020;**2**(3):1900105

[103] Hu X, Yasa IC, Ren Z, Goudu SR, Ceylan H, Hu W, et al. Magnetic soft micromachines made of linked microactuator networks. Science Advances. 2021;**7**(23):eabe8436

[104] Huebsch N, Kearney CJ, Zhao X, Kim J, Cezar CA, Suo Z, et al. Ultrasound-triggered disruption and self-healing of reversibly cross-linked

hydrogels for drug delivery and enhanced chemotherapy. National Academy of Sciences of the United States of America. 2014;**111**(27):9762-9767

[105] Alford A, Tucker B, Kozlovskaya V, Chen J, Gupta N, Caviedes R, et al. Encapsulation and ultrasound-triggered release of G-quadruplex DNA in multilayer hydrogel microcapsules. Polymers. 2018;**10**(12):1342

[106] Xia S, Zhang Q, Song S, Duan L, Gao G. Bioinspired dynamic cross-linking hydrogel sensors with skin-like strain and pressure sensing behaviors. Chemistry of Materials. 2019;**31**(22):9522-9531

[107] Zhu T, Cheng Y, Cao C, Mao J, Li L, Huang J, et al. A semi-interpenetrating network ionic hydrogel for strain sensing with high sensitivity, large strain range, and stable cycle performance. Chemical Engineering Journal. 2020;**385**:123912

[108] Alvarez MP, Burrezo PM, Iwamoto T, Qiu L, Kertesz M, Taravillo M, et al. Chameleon-like behaviour of cyclo [n] paraphenylenes in complexes with C 70: On their impressive electronic and structural adaptability as probed by Raman spectroscopy. Faraday Discussions. 2014;**173**:157-171

[109] Yu J, Wang J, Zhang Y, Chen G, Mao W, Ye Y, et al. Glucose-responsive insulin patch for the regulation of blood glucose in mice and minipigs. Nature Biomedical Engineering. 2020;**4**(5):499-506

[110] Tong MQ, Luo LZ, Xue PP, Han YH, Wang LF, Zhuge DL, et al. Glucose-responsive hydrogel enhances the preventive effect of insulin and liraglutide on diabetic nephropathy of rats. Acta Biomaterialia. 2021;**122**:111-132

[111] Liu HY, Greene T, Lin TY, Dawes CS, Korc M, Lin CC. Enzyme-mediated stiffening hydrogels for probing activation of pancreatic stellate cells. Acta Biomaterialia. 2017;**48**:258-269

[112] Liu HY, Korc M, Lin CC. Biomimetic and enzyme- responsive dynamic hydrogels for studying cell-matrix interactions in pancreatic ductal adenocarcinoma. Biomaterials. 2018;**160**:24-36

[113] Souza SF, Silva ER, Alves WA. Nanostructured antigen-responsive hydrogels based on peptides for leishmaniasis detection. Journal of the Brazilian Chemical Society. 2017;**28**:1619-1629

[114] Lim SL, Ooi CW, Tan WS, Chan ES, Ho KL, Tey BT. Biosensing of hepatitis B antigen with poly (acrylic acid) hydrogel immobilized with antigens and antibodies. Sensors and Actuators B: Chemical. 2017;**252**:409-417

[115] Gholamali I. Stimuli-responsive polysaccharide hydrogels for biomedical applications: A review. Regenerative Engineering and Translational Medicine. 2021;**7**:91-114

[116] Liang X, Wang X, Xu Q, Lu Y, Zhang Y, Xia H, et al. Rubbery chitosan/carrageenan hydrogels constructed through an electroneutrality system and their potential application as cartilage scaffolds. Biomacromolecules. 2018;**19**(2):340-352

[117] da Silva SB, Krolicka M, van den Broek LA, Frissen AE, Boeriu CG. Water-soluble chitosan derivatives and pH-responsive hydrogels by selective C-6 oxidation mediated by TEMPO-laccase redox system. Carbohydrate Polymers. 2018;**186**:299-309

[118] Leu HY, Farhoudi N, Reiche CF, Koerner J, Mohanty SK, Solzbacher F, et al. Low-cost microfluidic sensors with smart hydrogel patterned arrays using electronic resistive channel sensing for readout. United States patent application US 16/601,120. 2020

[119] Liu L, Yao W, Rao Y, Lu X, Gao J. pH-responsive carriers for oral drug delivery: Challenges and opportunities of current platforms. Drug Delivery. 2017;**24**(1):569-581

[120] Xiang T, Lu T, Zhao WF, Zhao CS. Ionic-strength responsive zwitterionic copolymer hydrogels with tunable swelling and adsorption behaviors. Langmuir. 2018;**35**(5):1146-1155

[121] Andrade F, Roca-Melendres MM, Durán-Lara EF, Rafael D, Schwartz S Jr. Stimuli-responsive hydrogels for cancer treatment: The role of pH, light, ionic strength and magnetic field. Cancers. 2021;**13**(5):1164

[122] Samchenko Y, Ulberg Z, Korotych O. Multipurpose smart hydrogel systems. Advances in Colloid and Interface Science. 2011;**168**(1-2):247-262

[123] Lim HL, Hwang Y, Kar M, Varghese S. Smart hydrogels as functional biomimetic systems. Biomaterials Science. 2014;**2**(5):603-618

[124] Wang Z, Hu Y, Xue Y, Zhu Z, Wu Y, Zeng Q, et al. Mechanism insight on licorice flavonoids release from carbopol hydrogels: Role of "release steric hindrance" and drug solubility in the release medium. European Journal of Pharmaceutical Sciences. 2022;**179**:106307

[125] Chen Y, Wang X, Tao S, Wang Q, Ma PQ, Li ZB, et al. Research advances in smart responsive-hydrogel dressings with potential clinical diabetic wound healing properties. Military Medical Research. 2023;**10**(1):37

[126] Samiraninezhad N, Asadi K, Rezazadeh H, Gholami A. Using chitosan, hyaluronic acid, alginate, and gelatin-based smart biological hydrogels for drug delivery in oral mucosal lesions: A review. International Journal of Biological Macromolecules. 2023;**252**:126573

[127] Wang X, Luan F, Yue H, Song C, Wang S, Feng J, et al. Recent advances of smart materials for ocular drug delivery. Advanced Drug Delivery Reviews. 2023;**200**:115006

[128] Salehi S, Naghib SM, Garshasbi HR, Ghorbanzadeh S, Zhang W. Smart stimuli-responsive injectable gels and hydrogels for drug delivery and tissue engineering applications: A review. Frontiers in Bioengineering and Biotechnology. 2023;**11**:1104126

[129] Zhou C, Wu T, Xie X, Song G, Ma X, Mu Q, et al. Advances and challenges in conductive hydrogels: From properties to applications. European Polymer Journal. 2022;**177**:111454